Chiropractic Revolution

Why Chiropractic Care is on the Rise

I0067680

Seven Falls Publishing

Chiropractic Revolution

Why Chiropractic Care Is On the Rise

Andy R. Curry

The publisher of this book is generously donating all royalties from the retail sales of "**CHIROPRACTIC REVOLUTION**" to:

St. Jude Children's Research Hospital

The mission of St. Jude Children's Research Hospital is to advance cures, and means of prevention, for pediatric catastrophic diseases through research and treatment. Consistent with the vision of founder Danny Thomas, no child is denied treatment based on race, religion or family's ability to pay.

You can learn more about
St. Jude Children's Research Hospital by visiting
www.stjude.org

This book was made possible by tips from the following:

Dr. Victor Poletajev

Dr. Allison Ross

Dr. Ray Nannis

Dr. Hong Yim

Dr. Dan Lavanga

Dr. Steven Buras

Dr. Phillip Reyes

Dr. Bradley Mouroux

Dr. Doreen Lewis

Dr. Morgan Oaks

Dr. Chris Michlin

Dr. Andrew Waitkevich

Dr. Mitchell Pearce

Dr. Jason Kramer

Dr. Amber Bloom

CONTENTS

FORWARD..10

CHAPTER ONE...12
Dr. Victor Poletajev
   Accident and Wellness Care Center

CHAPTER TWO..35
Dr. Allison Ross
   Ross Chiropractic

CHAPTER THREE...45
Dr. Ray Nannis
   Optimum Wellness Solutions

CHAPTER FOUR...61
Dr. Hong Yim
   Horizon Wellness Center Inc.

CHAPTER FIVE...74
Dr. Dan Lavanga

Lavanga Holistic Center

CHAPTER SIX………………………………………..86

Dr.Steven Buras

Jones Road Chiropractic

CHAPTER SEVEN…………………………………...97

Dr. Phillip Reyes

Clinton Chiropractic

CHAPTER EIGHT………………………………….…..107

Dr. Bradley Mouroux

Mouroux Chiropractic

CHAPTER NINE……………………………………119

Dr. Doreen Lewis

San Pedro North Chiropractic

CHAPTER TEN……………………..………………129

Dr. Morgan Oaks

An Evolution in Chiropractic

CHAPTER ELEVEN………………..………………143

Dr. Chris Michlin

CHAPTER TWELVE..161
Dr. Andrew Waitkevich

CHAPTER THIRTEEN....................................170
Dr. Mitchell Pearce

CHAPTER FOURTEEN...................................190
Dr. Jason Kramer

CHAPTER FIFTEEN......................................204
Dr. Amber Bloom

FOREWARD

As I interviewed these doctors of chiropractic, I was introduced to a world of healthcare that was much deeper and special than I already knew.

You see, the general consensus out there is that chiropractors are back crackers. This comes from the noise made when a spine is adjusted. Frankly, the word "crack" has a connotation of pain and/or danger. Yet chiropractic is one of the safest health practices. It's unfortunate that the assumption exists because chiropractic has been around for a long time and the health benefits are amazing. People go to chiropractors for back and neck pain, but also for wellness.

There have been astonishing events that have occurred from chiropractic. For instance, patients have often left a treatment seeing colors more vividly and brightly. There have been folks treated for asthma with chiropractic and found relief anywhere from slight to significant. Many have been treated for migraines. The level of relief found has often been tremendous.

In fact, you would be surprised about the number issues chiropractic can address. My suggestion is to read through these interviews to get a feel for what is possible. I promise you will be surprised by the health benefits. Once you get a feel for that and you find you have an issue you need help with, see if you can find a chiropractor to help you. You might be delightfully surprised at the results.

I also want you to look over the myths and misconceptions revealed by the interviewed doctors. As you read them, you may see yourself thinking the same thing. For example, one myth is there is no science behind chiropractic. Yet, there is a lot of research done by spine and disc specialists, physical therapists, and yes, medical doctors.

It may surprise you to know there are more than 200 different specialties, techniques, and emphasis that can be treated with chiropractic. It can range from nutrition to neurology and energy balancing, energy work, and more. What's important is you know all chiropractors are different. As you search for one that works for you, hang on to them because you may never find another like them.

CHAPTER ONE

DR. VICTOR POLETAJEV

ACCIDENT AND WELLNESSCARE CENTER

DR. VICTOR POLETAJEV

Dr. Victor Poletajev is a board certified chiropractic physician with a practice that specializes in accident and injury care, nutrition, and physical assessment. He holds five state licenses, performs independent medical examinations and testimony in Tennessee, West Virginia, Pennsylvania, Delaware, and Alabama. He is board certified in impairment and disability evaluations with certificates by ABIME, AADEP, ABFP, and ABDA. He has over 110 hours of post-graduate education in forensic impairment and disability evaluations alone. He has performed over 5900 plus, third party, independent medical evaluations, including Workers' Compensation, Social Security Disability, Personal Injury, Veteran's Administration and, consulting for National Football League Disability claims. He has been deposed 180 plus times in twenty years of experience.

Dr. Poletajev is published in the areas of sports injury, rehabilitation, and nutrition in magazines such as Muscle AND Fitness and Power lifting, USA. He was an appointed team physician for the Natural Association of Strength Athletes for eight years and worked with other organizations like the A.A.U. and the U.S.P.F.

Dr. Poletajev is fluent in Russian language, and has completed hundreds of hours of post-graduate training in motor vehicle accident injury, sports injury, nutrition, diagnosis, activities of daily living, pain relief, and wellness care and assessment.

Dr. Poletajev orders MRI studies on a regular basis to verify and substantiate his findings as well as when treating. In the practice of independent medical examinations, history, causation, reasonableness, and necessity of standards of care are all addressed. Dr. Poletajev was an appointed complaint consultant for the board for five years in Tennessee.

Dr. Poletajev has examined, rated, and treated from muscular-skeletal conditions, conditions such as sprain strains, surgical fusion, discectomy, amputation, extremity conditions, including joint replacement, i.e. knee, shoulder, also including burn victims, scarring, RSD, nerve entrapment, carpal tunnel, and stroke with organic brain syndrome, as well as quadriplegics, including expectant mothers.

Dr. Poletajev brings to his expert testimony as well as practice as represented in deposition and court situations, simple explanations, authoritative representation of the 4th, 5th and 6th edition AMA Guides, when required, and makes himself available for plaintiff and defense consultation within his area of expertise. He has obtained, successfully, as an expert, in regards to his independent examinations, for and against specialties including internal medicine, psychiatry, neurology, orthopedic, dermatology, osteopathic and chiropractic physicians. In independent examinations he is methodical, explained, well-footnoted, strictly following the criteria parameter protocol of both state statues, various jurisdictional law and of course the AMA guides.

Dr. Poletajev has been to trial court as an expert and due to his detail-oriented and precise independent examinations, court exposure and adversarial action is minimized.

Conversation with Dr. Poletajev:

Question: Please tell us about your practice and the patients you serve.

Dr. Poletajev: My name is Victor Poletajev, D.C. The D.C. behind my name is for doctor of chiropractic. I currently practice in Murfreesboro, Tennessee. My practice specializes in restoring athletes and increasing abilities to perform daily activities-functional medicine and pain relief. Most people don't understand what a chiropractic doctor is and a lot of people have heard myths about chiropractic that have made them a little skeptical. It's interesting to note that "form follows function".

The fact is that the body has certain types of biological and physiological functions. Research has taken bodies of different animals and put perfectly healthy joints in plaster. After four to six weeks, when they removed those joints from plaster, they found that those joints had fused and become restricted. That should give you an instant mental picture of how important preserving range of motion is and how this affects your daily activities. This is typically why people seek physicians who understand biomechanical function and kinetic action. Yes, there is such a practitioner and he's known as a doctor of chiropractic medicine.

How did chiropractic come to be? In this country, it's a little over 110 years old. It was founded by Dr. Daniel David Palmer of Davenport, Iowa. He was the first to call himself a chiropractor in Greek, "done by hand". Chiropractic is based off of Chinese medicine, which is over 5000 years old. Care of this type is billed under physical medicine modalities and that's what a chiropractic physician would bill in the CPT codebook. In the medical model, we are practitioners of physical medicine. Dr. David Palmer, who started the first chiropractic school, Palmer College of Chiropractic, actually discovered this through oriental medicine. Dr. Palmer believed in the state of, "Dis Ease": the fundamental ability of the nerve interference to be corrected through spinal manipulation that would help the body correct the condition. Dr. Palmer treated all organic and non-organic conditions with manipulation. Over the years, chiropractic faced difficulty in acceptance because the chiropractic doctor was viewed as a medical doctor and he's not. He's not a medical provider. He does not prescribe medicine or only deal with symptoms. The chiropractor is the restorer of form and function-getting the human form to adapt back to full function and/or restore as much as possible.

When Dr. Palmer started the first school, he had a deaf patient named Harvey Willard. Dr. Palmer is credited with restoring his hearing. It's not magic. It's not mystical. It's anatomical. In chiropractic, we typically get patients that have exhausted all forms of medical treatment and/or athletes that use their bodies in extraordinary ways, who push themselves and want to get maximum movement. I call this homeostatic movement.

The chiropractic adjustment is a correction everybody will benefit from. You're trying to get the most use out of your body, whether you realize it or not, and that's why you're seeking the chiropractor. Obviously a pill in a bottle is not going to solve an actual mechanical problem. This is why NSAIDs have been proven to have little to no effect with, let's say, back pain or neck pain.

Research revealed that the first episode of back pain usually resolves itself within six weeks without a whole lot of to-do. The problem is that now you have healed the joint tissue in a compromised pattern. You have not restored your range of motion, so you can expect a second, third, fourth, and maybe a fifth or sixth episode of back pain. Those are not going to be as forgiving and ultimately, the person will end up in increased pain scenario that lands them in our office. Patients mostly find us on the insurance provider list because chiropractic is accepted in all states. Most insurance companies reimburse for chiropractic. Chiropractic physicians are one of the three physicians, according to Medicare. We also receive medical referrals.

Researchers in the early 90s introduced a study on chiropractic adjustments and sports. They took perfectly healthy athletes and placed them in two groups. They had a sham group, meaning they took half the group and they gave them sham chiropractic adjustments, and the other group got six weeks of chiropractic adjustments. Prior to the study, they assessed them in biometrics, jumping, running, agility, and sports drills. After six weeks, the group that had the chiropractic adjustments had a 10-15% increase in function. These were asymptomatic patients; they did not have back pain or neck pain to begin with. These perfectly healthy individuals were just assessed. Of course the sham group didn't have an increase at all in testing.

There's another interesting study in foot orthotics; here they put participants in golf shoes and had them swing golf clubs. My daughter played professional junior golf all the way up to college and a lot of athletes feel more comfortable and they're able to hit the ball better in orthotics. The results of this study showed that when the individuals balanced in the foot orthotics, their club head speed increased up to 15%.

This is all bio mechanical function and restoration. I know I'm going a little bit further than just explaining, but with a chiropractic adjustment, we can actually balance the proprioception, resulting in things like increased comfort and club speed. Proprioception is a big word, but it is simply the joints' ability to sense its position in space and time. To increase the proprioception, it requires a correction to the mechanoreceptors that send a message to the brain through tracts. I know that's a little much, but that's what we do.

We restore dysfunctional tissue in multiple ways. We have physiological therapeutics where we administer different methods like laser, ultrasound, Russian muscles stem, and micro current. We video and observe kinetic motion with athletes and also perform dry needle. After forty years of weight training and a competitive lifting career, I offer personal training with an adaptive formula that increases physical fitness and function without aggravating injured joints. I restore the body to full function and strength. I order blood chemistries and correct weight with nutrition from my own vitamin line, Myostar ™. I have treated men and women with conditions where they feel terrible and tired. After the blood values are recorded, we correct the indices and the patients respond. They regain their lives and are grateful. Recently, I had a female patient who was tired and had irritable bowel syndrome. After three weeks of care she confided that she was off all of her medicines for colitis and had never felt so good.

In my practice specifically, I've gotten involved with independent medical exams. Independent medical exams are where somebody requires a physician to come in and examine them as a third party. These are not patients of mine. These are other patients that are either sent to me from an attorney or another source, like a chiropractic doctor or another medical provider. They want me to ascertain their basic restrictions and limitations. I am ABIME certified, American Board of Independent Medical Examiners. I have been for years and I have other certificates in that area of expertise by the American Academy of Evaluating Physicians, American Board of Forensic Professionals, and the American Board of Disability Analysts. A total of four Board certificates. In my practice, I've performed over 5,800 independent medical exams consisting of Veteran's claims, Worker's Compensation, Social Security, and personal injury claims. What this has done is honed my diagnostic skills. Meeting somebody on a one-time basis, I have to figure out what's going on with their body, what's wrong with them, and make sure the diagnosis is appropriate.

With all of that, it's pretty information intense, and has helped me pinpoint my skills to determine a condition. Most chiropractic physicians do not get involved with medical examinations due to the labor intensity. Court testimony is associated with this field of endeavor and this to may create a hindrance. I first started medical examinations years ago in West Virginia treating nothing but injury, injury, injury. I ended up doing exams because I was asked by a UMWA official to perform medical examinations on injured coal miners.

This has helped me with my ability to make a proper diagnosis and if needed, I have test privileges in hospitals. This is valuable in coming up with a treatment, and examining a patient or client for a third party. Now days, a lot of people are running around with conditions and there are so many diseases out there that are new, so it's important to get a proper diagnosis and make sure that the diagnosis fits your treatment. We're very specific about that. It's not one size fits all. The body's dynamic and when you're treating people; everybody's a little bit different and there's a lot of overlapping factors that determine a person's diagnosis and the type of treatment they're going to receive.

A lot of people are resistant to chiropractic care when they first hear about it simply because they do not know what chiropractors do or how effective it is. In chiropractic medicine, we treat scoliosis with adjustments and measurements. Medicine surgical treatment requires fusion with rods and eventually down the road, it causes organic fusion. When the rods are removed, the person has lost a lot of range of motion, kinetics sense, and their proprioception with the spinal joints. You can see how this is very bad. Now, they're basically an old person at a young age. With no motion, the spine deteriorates and is rigid.

With this nonsurgical correction, we preserve motion and have documented outcomes. What we do and we're very, very specific, is adjust in the scoliotic convexity area. Convexity is the outer portion where the C curve is located.

We adjust into that to make a correction. Anatomically, you can measure a child or young adult let's say six, seven, and eight. You can have a different leg length, an anatomical leg length for each year or each six months possibly of gestation and what happens is you have this person that's actually growing unbalanced. Now, you put in the pressures of sports or a fifty-pound backpack. This combination is the perfect and it doesn't help that backpacks are the number two reason for the ER visits in this age range. People don't realize that when school's in session. The children develop back pain and of course the parents think that they're too young for back pain. No, they can have back pain. What happens is they develop scoliosis. We offer a scoliotic assessment and if necessary, we order x-rays and go over the plan of attack.

Chiropractic is statistically very safe. Our malpractice rate is extremely low. Currently, there are about 60,000 practicing chiropractors in the United States and when I was at Palmer completing my internship for my chiropractic degree, there were four clinics. Visits were in the millions of adjustments per year. One year it went up to about seven million. There were only 250,000 residents in the Quad City area. We used to comment how we were all well adjusted there. There were also hundreds of chiropractic physicians' clinics in the QC area. With all those adjustments, we never heard of any irontogenic reactions to care aka a bad reaction to chiropractic treatment. They've done all kinds of studies and chiropractic care is very safe. We have extensive class hours, didactic class hours, and intern rounds. A licensed doctor of chiropractic medicine completes a four-year undergrad with a three and a half year chiropractic college.

Years ago, chiropractic was considered something that was quasi medicine and there was even a short time where chiropractic was covered in the American Medical Association's committee on Quackery. The Wilk trial. Dr. Wilk was a chiropractic physician and he discovered through his own investigations, that the AMA was actually pumping money into their system to contain and eliminate chiropractic. They didn't want the competition for patients. This actually went to court. Dr. Wilk's brother, George, was an attorney and represented the case. The AMA was found guilty of subversion and trying to eliminate chiropractic. They also lost the appeal in the Supreme Court. They had to pay restitution back to the chiropractic profession. This was concluded in the 80s. Not many people know about it. The AMA had to cease and desist and re-write that it was ethical to refer to chiropractic physicians.

I've had medical physicians as patients over the years. They come from a different philosophy. They believe that with medicine the body will correct itself. Unfortunately, with a mechanical problem, the body has shown to have almost no response but a short-lived pain decrease. In medical research, and the advent of the physiology of the adjustment, the medical community realized it's not "voodoo" anymore. Now the other profusions are less skeptical of chiropractic.

I actually looked into becoming a doctor of osteopathic medicine. This was back in the early 80s. I applied to PCOM-Philadelphia College of Osteopathic Medicine. When I applied there, I was interested in physical medicine. I had this idea, which probably was considered crazy at that time, of treating nonsurgical and rehabbing sports injuries. When I looked at PCOM, they had no physical medicine. They didn't even do manipulation.

In osteopathic medicine, they believe that the adjustment is a long lever adjustment. They believed adjustment affected the arterial and the venous system versus the chiropractic profession that believed affects neurology. In 1955, the osteopaths had to give up their philosophy on adjusting and obtained a prescription pad.

It's interesting to note now that the osteopaths are trying to reintroduce some of that manipulation into their schools because of all the research the chiropractic profession has done on manipulation. They're realizing how effective that manipulation is for, not just musculoskeletal things, but things like blood pressure and other conditions.

In the 1990s there was a study by Dr. Eddy, an MD/PhD at Duke University. Dr. Eddy was trying to discover what percentage of medical treatment is scientifically based. He decided it was 15%. That blew people away. The thing is that doctor basically means learned person and practice is practice. We're all practicing. You never know what's going to walk in your office. People are dynamic. They bring different situations and scenarios to the clinic.

I was an athlete. I did Olympic lifting, which is now called weightlifting. Back then there was one person maybe in my whole school that participated in the sport and maybe two others in the entire area. It really was not very popular. I competed and was a Junior Olympics Champion. I qualified, placed 2nd one year and I actually won the Junior Olympics in weightlifting for my weight category in 1976. Then, I had an injury. I detached my triceps tendon and I had an avulsion tear of my left ulna. This required surgery. I had two surgical procedures. After that, I was still able to compete and qualified for the 1980 Olympics. We didn't go in 1980, but I had more injuries and that limited my lifting.

I also competed in power lifting, a different weight sport. I ended up winning some state and national titles and I still hold a National and Junior World Record for the bench press. I bench pressed 245 kilos or 540 pounds and that was in 1981. That's the only record I still hold. I tore a pectorals muscle in 1982 and I was the only lifter to ever get close to my best lifts after surgical correction.

With my background, I thought and deliberated extensively about the best way to treat sports injuries. I figured since medicine had nothing for nonsurgical sport injuries, chiropractic was a perfect fit. Well, chiropractic wasn't ready for me. When I went to school in 1982, I wanted to apply therapy, exercise, stretching, muscle work, and rehab to care, but they just weren't ready. Chiropractic school was solely teaching people to adjust at that point. I visited three different chiropractic schools and they were not doing sports treatment, it was basic adjustments.

My alma mater now teaches the same protocol I had put together in my clinic. My idea was to implement sports rehab and to bring it full circle with all the physical medicine modalities. We had ultrasound, muscle stim, exercise, and rehab stuff like teaching people how to sit on a gym ball and strengthening their backs. That's always been the premise of my treatment, to not only get the patient out of pain, but also get their back strong, and to get that core strengthened up.

At my clinic we have a complete rehab facility. It's basically a gym. I bring people back to function and suggest techniques that will work around their conditions. True functional medicine. Athletes that I have treated in the past-Olympians and pros alike-are focused and can benefit greatly. We specialize in a minimum amount of care and a quick recovery. I have rehabbed both shoulders and backs post-surgery.

Chiropractic has come full circle. They have a chiropractic physician for every NFL team. Then there are all your collegiate teams and even high schools are starting to employ chiropractic physicians.

Now there's buzz in medicine about preventative health care; chiropractic has been practicing preventive and functional medicine for years. In 1986, we had a treatment protocol for fibromyalgia. That was considered "voodoo" by medicine. It didn't exist. There was no blood test for fibromyalgia. Most people don't realize that a chiropractic physician is taught to do blood work. We order blood work and we monitor nutrition. We were the original nutrition doctors because there was no nutritional ND, nutritional doctorate. There were dietitians who were limited and PT's that had to go to a hospital or different homes for visitation. They weren't doing any kind of sports treatments. Massage, I don't want to say anything bad about the profession, massage is a wonderful thing, but back in the sixties and seventies, massage wasn't exactly something that people actually looked for or viewed as therapeutic. Now everything's come full circle.

Question: Do you have any patients that you would consider miraculous post treatment?

Dr. Poletajev: I've had all kinds of patients over the years; I've had children that I've adjusted and over a period of time, their asthma went away. I've had colleagues where I've actually given them an adjustment and their hearing was restored. I'm sure there's more than that from what I recall. We'll just keep it at this.

There's something important I want to mention. I was the only athlete to ever come back and actually do a bench press close to what I did before as a record after a pec tear. I tore my pec in 1982. I required surgery. That all stemmed from the fact that I had a football injury in 7th grade where I had broken the humerus in the growth plate. When I broke the humerus, my arm was set up for advanced degenerative changes in my left shoulder. Most people don't know that about me.

Every orthopedic surgeon that I ever went to couldn't believe I lifted what I did. It shouldn't be possible; I should not be able to do all that. Ultimately, I paid the price because my biomechanical motion was incorrect on that left side and it ended up tearing my pec. I had corrective surgery and I was able to come back and bench over 500 pounds again. I'm the only strength athlete to ever do that, the only one.

The fact is, these aren't really miracles. What they are is anatomical neurological stories. This is all anatomy. A chiropractic adjustment affects neurology. You can prove increased MCV ENG tests with a chiropractic adjustment. I've had people correct downgrade reflexes. It's not a miracle. We affect neurology of the bodies. What happens with a chiropractic adjustment? I tell patients this: It's kind of like when your computer is running really sluggish. You have all these viruses and the cookies are jamming up your computer. What do you do? You clean out the cookies; you reboot the computer, and clean it up. That's kind of what chiropractic adjustment does to the neurology of the body. It's very much like rebooting a computer.

I also see this lot now, a 350-pound plus patient with no exercise. I do blood work. I see indices that are skewed. We can correct those through nutrition and we do. Then when we start working on their bodies as far as giving them an exercise program; we give them some chiropractic treatment, and physical medicine modalities, and they improve. We can get their exercise level, and their cardiac output up, and everything changes. They start to feel better, they start to do better. Chiropractic, offers a different approach to than simply running for a pill and developing dependency on medication. We don't offer medicine; we offer a functional correction to these problems. These are not miracles; we're affecting the neurology of the body.

In total, that's basically what a chiropractor does. You have heard old wives tales, that chiropractic is dangerous. These are all sorts of stories that have no scientific basis. People don't know the truth about chiropractic and yet they're hearing things, making excuses for themselves, and then they don't want to do anything about their pain.

I've adjusted infants; I've adjusted my own child when she was three days old. Manipulation is very safe if it's done properly. When I say properly, I mean by a licensed chiropractic physician. The fact of the matter is, it is a type of training that we get that is based on the human body, how the human body heals, and natural medicine healing treats. Like I said, it's all anatomy, physiology, and neurology. These miracles that you hear about, they are basically neurological corrections.

I do believe a faith background helps in healing. I've been involved a Sub-deacon in my Orthodox church for 27 years. I believe there's a strong correlation between prayer and healing. I don't push my personal beliefs, but I do see that those who have more of a belief system and prayer seem to do better than those who do not. Like I said, that's up to the person.

In closing, I've been in practice for 30 years. I graduated in October of 1986. I currently hold five state licenses. I'm registered on the National Registry of Certified Medical Examiners for the Federal Motor Carrier Safety Administration which is the DOT exam for the CDL license, required by bus drivers and tractor trailers, semi-truck operators. I'm also board certified by the American Board of Independent Medical Examiners of the American Academy of Disability Evaluating Physicians, the American College of Disability Medicine, the American Board of Forensics Professionals, the American Board of Disability Analysts, etc. I am also Mackenzie certified. I was one of the original certified strength and conditioning specialists.

I also worked as a team doctor and treated Olympic athletes. The last time I went to the Olympics, it was in Sochi and I worked with the Ukrainian team. I've taken many classes in cranial therapy, and endo-nasal technique, these are all non-surgical and work with the head. There's a lot of neurology in the palates and sinuses. I like to upgrade my techniques. Any new technologies inspire me to take a class or get a certification. If it helps my patient, I'm all about it. It's very important to keep current.

A chiropractor can be a portal of entry physician and not just for musculoskeletal conditions. In other countries, where they use socialized medicine like Denmark or Norway, they use chiropractic and a chiropractor as a primary along with the medical primary.

Question: What are some health benefits of using a chiropractor?

Dr. Poletajev: Back in 1990, I worked as a team physician at NASA, the Natural Athletes Strength Association, and United States Power lifting. I worked with the weight lifters. When you get to work as a team doctor and you're on call, it's interesting how people respond. Often they'll have some type of muscle condition. Everyone has seen the taping and stuff like that. The Kinesio tape was actually invented by a chiropractor. This is all biomechanical. That's why a chiropractor works so well when a person has an injury and pain medication is not an option. You need to get them back in the game and if it's possible, a chiropractor can do wonders.

Speaking of health benefits, I also own a trademark vitamin line. It's called the Myostar line. I've had this for years. I have quality control and use only American source ingredients. We used to sell wholesale and now we do more retail. Over the years, I've worn different hats in my practice and I've done different things. In seeing patients, I enjoy the challenge. I give my patients my full attention. I came up with a slogan of my own, kind of spin off of other slogans: I use integrity with the pursuit of excellence in patient care. I believe that sums up what we do in our office and how I live my life. I'm here to help.

Question: What made you decide to become a chiropractor?

Dr. Poletajev: I decided on chiropractic school due to the absence of physical medicine and manipulation in D.O. school. When I arrived at chiropractic school, they were not doing the sports treatment; it was basically adjustments and manipulation care for health conditions. I had this idea about treating sports injuries. I wanted to bring sports rehab full circle by including all the physical medicine modalities. We had ultrasound, muscle stim, and of course, the most important thing is exercise and rehab like teaching people how to sit on a gym ball and strengthen their backs, not just giving them an adjustment and sending them out the door. That's always been the premise of my treatment, to not only get you out of pain, but also get your back strong and strengthen your core.

I've tried to keep ahead of the curve as far as what's good for the human body and how to help patients. I've always kept the natural functional medicine premise in mind. If medicine is needed, of course there's always a referral. I have medical doctors, nurse practitioners, and surgeons that I refer to.

Question: How can someone find out more about your practice?

Dr. Poletajev: If you have any interests, concerns, or comments, we have six phone numbers and several web pages. You can contact us through our web page. You can email us. You can call. Phone numbers are listed on the web page. We see patients from all over the country.

I'm located in Murfreesboro, Tennessee, central time zone, 615 area code. You can call 867-7522 or 867-3288. Some of our websites are: accidentandwellnesscarecenter.com, myostar.com, and jurispro.com/victorpoletajev.

There's something important I want to mention. I was the only athlete to ever come back and do a bench press close to what I did before. I tore my pec in 1982. I required surgery. That all stemmed from the fact that I had a football injury in 7th grade where I actually had broken the humerus in the growth plate. When I broke the humerus, my arm actually was set up for advanced degenerative changes in my left shoulder. Most people don't know that about me.

Every orthopedic surgeon that I ever went to, they couldn't believe I lifted what I did. It shouldn't have been possible. Ultimately, I paid the price because my biomechanical motion was not correct on that left side and it ended up tearing my pec. I had corrective surgery and I was able to come back and bench over 500 pounds again. I'm the only strength athlete to ever do that, the only one. I want to iterate that because with training, will, and chiropractic guidance, so much is possible that was previously deemed impossible.

CHAPTER TWO

DR. ALLISON ROSS
ROSS CHIROPRACTIC

DR. ALLISON ROSS, DC

Dr. Allison Ross, DC is a Palmer West Chiropractic College graduate. She uses a "whole body approach" when taking care of her patients. By combining hands-ontechnique, physiotherapy procedures, and clinical nutritional counseling, Dr. Ross is able to help patients accelerate and/or maintain their journey to good health.

Ross Chiropractic is a family practice. David Campagna and Dr. Allison Ross work together as husband and wife to promote the natural health benefits of Chiropractic care. Chiropractic has been a healthcare practice for over 100 years, yet many people have misconceptions concerning chiropractic. It is our mission to educate people and share the true benefits of chiropractic care. Chiropractic helps promote the body's natural ability to heal itself by enhancing your nervous system. People of all ages can benefit from chiropractic and that is why we encourage whole families to come in for care. Chiropractic helps restore and maintain optimal health and is a great way to get well and stay well naturally.

Conversation with Dr. Ross:

Question: Tell us about your practice and the patients you serve.

Dr. Ross: I practice a diversified method of chiropractic, which allows me to cater to a vast range of patients. My patients range in age and complaints, from neck and back pain to headaches, migraines, scoliosis, muscle tension, auto accident injuries, carpal tunnel, joint pain and/or dysfunction, etc. I offer physical therapy modalities as well as chiropractic adjustment therapy. I offer massage therapy, manual therapy, myofascial release, trigger point therapy, etc. People come in suffering, but leave feeling much better after their chiropractic treatment.

Question: Is there one problem that you specialize in solving?

Dr. Ross: Yes, I specialize in treating neuro-musculoskeletal conditions. To explain how chiropractic helps these conditions, I need to discuss an important term called "subluxation" also known as "joint segmental dysfunction" and/or "misalignment." A subluxation is a misalignment of vertebrae or joint, which affects: the joint, the disc (if in the spine), the surrounding tissues (muscles and ligaments), and the nerve. A subluxation can trigger pain, numbness, tingling, stiffness, reduced joint motion, etc. When a gentle force, i.e. "an adjustment" is delivered to this subluxation, the joint's motion is restored, the area can begin to heal, and the nerve flow is enhanced.

Question: What difference does the treatment you provide make in their everyday lives?

Dr. Ross: I'm able to offer safe, gentle, hands-on therapy without drugs or surgery. By treating misalignments of the spine or joints, the body can heal more effectively. I encourage patients to do stretches and exercises to help reduce stress on their bodies. I help them to identify some of the things in their lives that may be contributing to their ailments. Many people's ailments stem from repetitive stress at work or at home, so I counsel them on proper ergonomics, exercise therapy, pillow supports when sitting or sleeping, and what they can do to help to prevent the injuries and improve their overall health.

Question: What made you decide to become a chiropractor?

Dr. Ross: I've been a chiropractic patient since I was an infant and my older sister is a chiropractor. When I was born, I had congenital hip dysplasia, where my hip joints were misaligned and dislocated. The treatment was braces to proximate the hip to the socket.

After the braces came off, my parents, who had been chiropractic patients themselves for years, brought me in for a spinal evaluation, and I was adjusted. Growing up, chiropractic was always a part of our lives. We went regularly to have our spinal check-ups and had adjustments when necessary.

I decided that I wanted to be a chiropractor as a teenager, after working in a chiropractic office. Helping

38

people alleviate or get rid of pain altogether with chiropractic care was a natural decision for me.

Question: Tell me something that a patient you've helped considers a miracle.

Dr. Ross: I see little miracles every day when people come in with pain and leave with relief. One patient does come to mind, a woman who was suffering from migraines for years. The migraines were so debilitating that it affected every aspect of her life. With chiropractic care, we were able to reduce her migraines to the point that they were rare and infrequent.

It was incredible, how life changing that was for her, and for many other people who live with some form of pain or discomfort on a regular basis. Many people think their only form of treatment is pain medication, and that's simply not true. Chiropractic can help such a wide range of musculoskeletal conditions like neck and back pain, headaches, TMJ dysfunction, sciatica, joint pain, sports injuries, auto accident injuries, etc.

Question: Can you share a lesson you learned early on that still impacts how you run your practice today?

Dr. Ross: I take the time to get to know my patients. I treat them like family. Getting to know them helps me understand how their ailments manifest and learn what their goals are. For instance, if a patient loves gardening, but gardening triggers back pain, then we can set a goal to get back to gardening pain free.

Question: There are plenty of health benefits of using a chiropractor. Can you talk about that?

Dr. Ross: There are so many benefits to chiropractic. Obviously, number one is getting a person out of pain, two is to restore function, and three is to enhance that person's overall wellbeing through wellness care.

Question: Do you find that a lot of patients come back to you for regular adjustments as part of their health regiment?

Dr. Ross: Yes, everyone is under some form of stress nowadays, whether it is from work, home, or even physical strain from exercise. Chiropractic care reduces that stress on our bodies. This helps to enhance performance and vitality, thereby helping people reaches their health goals.

It's important that people understand the longer they wait for treatment, the harder it is to treat the problem. My patients experience firsthand, how an adjustment can provide, in many cases, instant relief and get them back to the activities they love as quickly as possible.

Question: What are some myths and misconceptions people generally have about chiropractic?

Dr. Ross: One that comes to mind is that once you have an adjustment, or once you start chiropractic care, that you'll always need it. How I address this question or this myth is with an example: You can't just exercise one day and expect to be fit for the rest of your life.

It is something that's ongoing. We will always have stress on our bodies, whether it is from sleeping the wrong way or working long hours on the computer without any breaks. That stress on our bodies impacts our vital health. It is important to come in, get your spinal alignment checked, and get adjusted to reduce that stress on your body.

Question: What are some common fears people have about chiropractic?

Dr. Ross: I would say the most common one is that the adjustment will hurt. I practice a diversified method of adjustment therapy; therefore I have many different ways of adjusting. I go through a thorough exam and screening with every patient, so that I can determine the safest, most effective method of treatment for each individual. For instance, if a patient is not comfortable with a manual cervical adjustment, then I would find an alternative method. I work with each individual's comfort level in order to make adjustments as gentle, and effective as possible.

Question: Does anybody ever ask you about side effects after an adjustment?

Dr. Ross: It is normal for there to be one of three things after an adjustment: one is that you feel great. You feel like the joint mobility and range of motion has improved, allowing you to move more freely and with less pain. Another possibility is that you don't feel a change immediately; that doesn't mean there isn't a change on a physiological level. Third is that there can be discomfort afterwards.

To explain the possibility of discomfort, I use the analogy of doing any strenuous exercise that your body is not used to, the body is sore afterwards. All three things are normal after an adjustment, but the most common is feeling pain relief.

Question: Describe a situation where you helped a patient overcome at least one misconception, fear, or unknown pitfall to help them feel better. What did you do?

Dr. Ross: When this happens, I do my best to fully explain everything that I am doing and why. If they are uncomfortable with getting, for instance, a manual cervical (neck) adjustment, I would never force them to have it. That's the advantage of being a diversified chiropractor; I have many different modalities, and techniques that can be used to accomplish my treatment goal. For example, I could use an activator.

Question: Would you describe what an activator is?

Dr. Ross: An activator is a hand-held adjustment instrument that delivers a low force to the joint, which helps restore mobility. The activator is virtually painless, and effective at adjusting. It has a variety of settings for different areas of the body, from very low force to a higher force. The lower back would need a higher force than say, the cervical (neck) area. It makes a clicking sound, and delivers the force to the joint, which helps to restore mobility.

Question: What's the one thing we haven't covered that you wish to share with someone who is considering chiropractic?

Dr. Ross: Schedule an appointment with a chiropractor to find out how they can help to improve your spinal health. A spinal check-up is very important; it helps to detect imbalances that can progressively worsen if left uncorrected. In other words, you shouldn't wait until something is broken to fix it. Go in and get a spinal checkup. A chiropractic evaluation may consist of a posture analysis, dual scales test, and range of motion testing, palpating muscle tone, spinal alignment, measuring BMI, blood pressure, gait analysis, or assessing foot imbalances.

If we catch these imbalances early on, in many cases we can save a person from developing neck or back pain, joint pain, plantar fasciitis, or a long list of conditions that people come in with. Chiropractic is beneficial for people of all ages. Like I said, I was an infant when I was first introduced to chiropractic.

If I could just spend a moment talking about pregnancy and the benefits of chiropractic care. Pregnancy, both labor and delivery puts an incredible strain on the spine, especially the low back. Many women with low back pain had their first episode of pain during or after pregnancy. By treating women during and after pregnancy, there's immediate pain relief and a better chance of preventing chronic back pain years later. Proper footwear is very important for spinal care as well. Unsupportive footwear can lead to foot problems like plantar fasciitis or low back pain.

Question: Have you done much work to help patients overcome plantar fasciitis?

Dr. Ross: Yes. I look at foot care quite a bit in my office. A lot of conditions in the low back, hips, knees, or upper back can stem from imbalances in the feet. There is a large portion of the population that is hyper pronated, which means flat-footed. Footwear, and foot care is essential to combating this issue and why I assess for foot imbalances. My goal is to educate patients on foot care, and effectively treat issues that spur from improper footwear.

Question: How can someone find out more about your practice?

Dr. Ross: My clinic name is Ross Chiropractic and we are located in San Jose, California. My website is www.drallisonrossdc.com. Our clinic phone number is 408-247-4503. Our address is 1142 South Winchester Boulevard in San Jose, California. Zip code 95128.

Dr. Ray Nannis

Optimum Wellness Solutions

Dr. Ray L. Nannis (Clinic Director/Owner) was born in Lawrence, Massachusetts on September 9, 1971. Dr. Nannis and his family moved to Richardson, Texas in 1977. His undergraduate work took place at Stephen F. Austin in Nacogdoches, Texas.

Dr. Nannis graduated from Parker College of Chiropractic (now Parker University) on September 11, 1995. He achieved a Bachelor of Science in Human Anatomy and Doctors of Chiropractic degrees.

Dr. Nannis furthered his education, and became a Fellow of the International Academy of Medical Acupuncture, a Master of Bioenergetics Synchronization Technique, and has studied over 25 chiropractic, and healing arts. He has a Reconnections level IV certification, has undergone extensive study in nutrition and emotional wellness, and is a Master in Holistic Psychology.

Dr. Nannis operated Nannis Chiropractic Family Health Center in East Richardson from 1997 to 2013. He later combined clinics with Harrington Chiropractic, and moved to West Richardson in 2013.

Dr. Nannis has spent his life heavily involved in the Richardson Community. His current activities include auto racing, and raising his daughters, Shelby and Sierra.

Conversation with Dr. Nannis:

Question: Tell us about your practice and the patients you serve.

Dr. Nannis: My practice is called Optimum Wellness Solutions. We are located in Richardson, Texas, which is immediately north of Dallas. I've been in practice for 20 years. The patients I serve are, for the most part, a wellness based practice. We do a variety of things. It's a lot broader than chiropractic alone. It has, of course, chiropractics a foundation, so we deal with what a lot of people might suspect chiropractors deal with. Everything from your general aches and pains to people that has had some serious challenges with something in their life. We also help people recover from allergies, stop smoking, deal with diabetes, thyroid problems, chronic health challenges, and aid them inquest for overall health, and wellness improvement.

Question: Is there anything that you specialize in solving?

Dr. Nannis: My biggest challenge in life is that we help with a little bit of everything. Not in any specific order, we have a functional medicine component to our practice where we help people with diabetes, thyroid problems, weight loss resistance, chronic fatigue, fibromyalgia, and pretty much anything that you can name along those lines. We have a detoxification program where we help people with brain fog or memory problems. We even help people with Alzheimer's and Parkinson's. We have an allergy service where we help people make allergies disappear. We eliminate all sorts of allergies; food allergies, environmental allergies, etc. We have nonsurgical spinal decompression, where we help people that have disk problems spanning from cervical disk problems to low back disk problems.

Obviously, we also do traditional chiropractic care where we help people with headaches, and such. There's not much I can't help one way or another.

Question: What do you do to help patients with fibromyalgia?

Dr. Nannis: Fibromyalgia is predominantly a nervous system problem, even though that's not in its name at all. The core component is a neurological approach to chiropractic care. What happens with fibromyalgia is that there's a problem in the mid brain where they're not getting enough stimulation from the body up to what's called the thalamus, which is kind of the grand central station of our brain. The input is where the challenge comes from. What happens is we have-usually it's some form of a loss of motion-a loss of input to the brain, and the lower part of the brainstem isn't getting the stimulation that it needs to stimulate the middle part of the brainstem. Then from that down regulation-that's what stops people from having the chronic aches and pains-everything just hurt all of the time.

Our first step in the battle against fibromyalgia is chiropractic care. A lot of times there are allergies associated with that, so we work with our allergy system to help ease some of the pain. Many times, there are some serious nutritional imbalances, so we work with that, as well. Other times, they are simply depleted of oxygen, and need a supplement. We can help provide oxygen to improve oxygenation of the body and the brain. It's a multifaceted approach. There's not one right answer. There's not a custom stamp that's going to fit everybody.

Question: What is your success rate for helping fibromyalgia patients?

Dr. Nannis: We have a tremendous success rate. I would say probably 90 to 95% of the people feel like they get their lives back.

Question: What made you decide to become a chiropractor?

Dr. Nannis: When I was about 11 years old or so, I rode around a lot in a truck with my stepfather. We had a landscape business, and every once in a while, he'd go into this office, and he'd come back feeling better. When I was about 14, my mother had a major slip and a fall, and she's a teacher, so she was not really capable of going back to work.

This happened close to the beginning of summer. She was flat on her back. She went to the M.D. She did everything they suggested, and she still could barely move. She was getting close to incapacitation. My stepfather, after a couple of months, drove her to his chiropractor, and within just a few visits, she was up and moving, and within a few weeks or a few months, she was pretty much back to normal.

That doctor had a Friends and Family Day. They brought me in and I got a checkup. We would have said I was a normal, healthy kid, but we did an exam, and the doctor said, "This kid's got some problems with his spine and we can fix them now. It'll be simpler and easier or we can wait until things break down further and he'll crawl into my office in 15 or 20 years." Fortunately, my parents decided to get my spine adjusted. I don't think I told him, but I had a headache every day of my life, literally 365 headaches a year, and relatively quickly they reduced to every other day, and within a few weeks, they were every third day, and within a couple more weeks after that, etc., I went from 365 headaches a year to about 12.

That wasn't enough to impress me, but after a few months in North Texas, allergy capital, I changed my mind. I had suffered from horrible allergies for as long as I could remember. We tried allergy medication. We basically tried everything. After about nine months, my mother asked if I needed more Sudafed and I told her I quit taking it. She said, "So, how are you breathing?" I said, "I don't know." The only thing that we could think of was that we had started chiropractic care.

I went to the chiropractor and asked him if there was anything he was doing that could have helped my allergies. He shared three things over the course of that visit; a book and a few other things. He said that the body is supposed to heal itself and any interference with that is called subluxation. That's what a chiropractor treats and if we remove the interference through adjustments, the body is designed to be self-healing and can begin self-regulating. I fell in love with the concept at 14 or 15 years old and knew that's what I wanted to be.

Question: What lesson did you learn early on that still impacts how you run your practice today?

Dr. Nannis: When I was relatively young in practice, I was worked as an associate doctor in another practice. I'd say what truly struck me was two or three things. Number one, I had this patient; he was actually a Worker's Comp patient who had fallen off a ladder, and injured himself. He went to a PT, and an M.D. They did enough rehab to send him back to work, but didn't fully recover. He was a door router. He put the designs in big, heavy wood doors. After he lifted something and he hurt himself again, he came to me.

The very first thing I told him was that it was going to take a lot of time to fix him because he was a mess. Obviously, he heard me better than I heard me, because after a couple of months of not seeing a lot of improvement, he said that he knew that chiropractic was the right course of treatment for him so we kept going, but it felt like, to me, we weren't making a lot of progress. I kept trying different treatments and even suggested sending him somewhere else. He said, "You told me in the beginning that this was going to take some time," and I was like, "Yeah, but it's taken some time now and we haven't made progress yet."

Really, quite a bit of time. I'm thinking like six, seven, or eight months passed, and it felt like we weren't making any improvement and then all of a sudden, something clicked, and he got his life back. He was capable of going back to work, but it took a lot of time. What I learned is that he had more faith in the fact that I told him that healing takes time, and that as long as we were removing interference, we were heading in the right direction, and that it's not just about how you feel today. It's about how your body's healing. I think he had bought into it more than I did.

The lesson that I learned there, quite simply, is that I have to listen to what I tell people, and believe it. We don't lose our health overnight. It takes time for degeneration to occur. It takes time for problems to manifest. We have multiple accidents, multiple injuries, we have multiple insults to the system, and if we give the body the right input and the things that it needs, it will recover.

The body will heal if we give it enough time.

Question: What are the health benefits of using a chiropractor?

Dr. Nannis: I think the biggest health benefit is that it makes a connection with different aspects of the body. We're a physical body, we're a chemical body, we're a mental body, we're an emotional body, we're a spiritual body, and a I think that what happens a lot of the time is that each of those bodies is doing its own thing. Chiropractic makes those all work together, so that we get the most that we can out of life.

I could list every symptom in the book: aches and pains, numbness, tingling, spasms, swelling, burning, cramping, weakness, in coordination, and we help with all of those. There's no doubt about that. We help with every organ in the body, because what it really boils down to is that the nervous system is our master system. It controls and coordinates everything in the body, and if there's interference between the brain and the body, whether it is to the muscle, bone, joint, and skin or whether it is to any one of the organs in the body, something is not going to work correctly. By removing interference, and allowing the body to have good communication with the brain, the greatest benefit is that the body is able to work the way that it's supposed to. We live in a toxic environment with a tremendous amount of emotional stress. We live in an environment where we've had physical trauma from the moment of birth forward, and chiropractic helps unwind that.

Question: What are myths and misconceptions people generally have about chiropractic?

Dr. Nannis: I'd say the first thing is that people think that once you start chiropractic, you have to do it forever. I would say that that's not necessarily true, although like anything else that's healthy, you have to do things on a consistent basis. There are phases of chiropractic care and people can chose to do as little or as much as they want to, but you won't continue to gain benefits. I don't think you'll ever lose the benefits that you've gained, but unless we remove the physical, chemical, and emotional stresses from life, we have to do things continuously work to maintain these benefits. Once you go to a gym, it doesn't mean you have to go forever, but if you want to maintain your physique, yes, you do.

If you start a diet, you don't have to be on it forever, but if you want to maintain a healthy system, then you do have to eat well. Chiropractic fits into that. Chiropractic is something that is generally good for most people, and to continue to gain benefits from it, you do need to stay engaged, but you don't have to. It's a choice, a choice to be healthy.

Many people say that chiropractic care is expensive. In comparison to what? If we're talking about taking a Tylenol, yeah, we cost more than taking a Tylenol, but on the flip side, the Tylenol does more damage than good, although it may cover up a symptom. Chiropractic is not about covering up symptoms, it's about helping people with their overall health, and wellness. I think that being under regular chiropractic care, the minimal investment that you could make, typically a year's worth of chiropractic costs less than a day in a hospital.

My daughter slipped and fell when she was three years old. She cut her head open. She looked like she had a concussion. She was certainly acting like it. We rushed her to the hospital, and when you bring a limp three-year-old into a hospital, they don't even ask your name. They put her on a CT scan. We got two CTs and stitched up. Fortunately, there was no concussion. I guess she was just tired or something, I don't know, probably really stressed out from getting knocked on the head. It was $9,000 of care...for stitches. Don't get me wrong, it was worth every penny. We ruled out the concussion. I'm very grateful that she didn't have one, but $9,000 for literally, seven or eight stitches, that's steep.

People think that chiropractors and medical doctors don't work together. We do different things. I think that there's a time and place for both. People need to understand that there are four types of medical care. There's emergency care, which is what I just explained I went through with my daughter. I think most people make their primary health decisions in an emergency room. It's a bad place to do long-term healthcare, because it's incredibly nerve wracking just being in an emergency room.

The second type of healthcare is disease-oriented care, and that's where a lot of people get involved with medical doctors. You want to talk about expensive? See how much a heart attack costs. See how much cancer costs. Ongoing treatment for those is insane, in the hundreds of thousands to millions of dollars sometimes. These are patients that have a definitive diagnosis, and they're getting a treatment for it. Sometimes it's short-term, sometimes it's long-term, either way, or the costs are astronomical.

The third type of healthcare is what I would call epigenetic care. Epigenetic care is where chiropractic fits in. It's about helping people and it's what my office does; it helps people look at their lifestyle, and make choices that help their body express optimum health and wellness, hence my name Optimum Wellness Solutions.

Then there's a fourth type of care that is called centropic care. Centropic care is about helping the body become more organized. We've got an incredible organization, because somehow or another, we took one cell, and became 700 trillion cells, and all of those cells work together for mutual benefit. That's under the coordination of the nervous system, and there are very few things that help organize that. I would say chiropractic is at the top of the list of what helps the body become more organized, simply because centropy is the opposite of entropy. The second law of thermodynamics basically says all things degenerate. They all degrade. They all break down, and the example that I always give is with my two-year-old and my three-year-old. Leave them alone in a toy room for just a few moments, and see what it looks like. Anybody with kids knows what I'm talking about. Leave a garden alone for a couple of weeks and your nice, neat rows are full of weeds, and the weeds take over, the plants don't.

Basically, anything that requires some form of order to become more organized requires a lot of energy.

Somehow or another, our bodies work very far from entropy, because we do become more organized. We go from one cell to 700 trillion cells and that's a very organized system, but what can happen is stress; physical, chemical, emotional stresses. Stress disorganizes those things. They move the body towards entropy, but by doing a few things, we can actually move the body back towards centropy, where we're reorganizing. We're becoming stronger. We're becoming more in order.

Chiropractic is a major component of maintaining organization. I think acupuncture help, too. I think Ayurvedic medicine does as well, but there aren't many things on the planet that truly do help the body become more organized or where the goal isn't just to get somebody over being sick, but to actually make you healthier for the next year. I'm 44 years old, and I will tell you that I'm healthier than I was when I was 14 because I've been under chiropractic care for 30 years.

A lot of people fear that chiropractic isn't safe. I would say that chiropractic is the safest thing on the planet as far as healthcare. If we look at the insurance rates, my next door neighbor was a medical doctor for a long time, and he was complaining about his malpractice insurance. He told me he was paying $25,000 a year for malpractice insurance as a general practitioner. I was surprised because my malpractice insurance costs less than my driving insurance. It costs me more to drive to work than to cover myself as a practitioner, and I carry the highest levels that a chiropractor is allowed. That just tells you that I'm safer as a chiropractor than a motorist.

Insurance companies are not losing money. They charge premiums where they make money. They're not losing anything, so you tell me who's safer. Thousands of people die every year in the numbers in the hundreds of thousands from incorrect prescriptions or correct prescriptions that went wrong. People die more from aspirin. Chiropractors are incredibly safe, but I will tell you that I think that there's some due diligence that needs to be done. Some chiropractors don't do it right; they don't give thorough exams to ensure that what they're doing is safe or get a comprehensive picture of what is going on.

I think chiropractors should be take x-rays of people's spines. They should perform thorough neurologic and orthopedic examinations. They should be do computer evaluations to find out what's happening with the nervous system, so that they know what they're working with. I think some of my colleagues look at chiropractic as a fancy bar trick, where we can lay someone down anywhere, and start working on his or her spine.

Question: What's one thing that we haven't covered that you'd like to share with someone who's considering chiropractic?

Dr. Nannis: The question that I would ask anybody is how important is their health? Because here's what I see: I see what happens as most people get older, they start to leave bits and pieces of their life behind. Whatever they enjoyed, whatever they found important in their life, whether that be playing with their children, being productive at work, bowling, golf or some other sport, what I see is people slowly leave little bits themselves behind as they travel down the road of life. Usually, this is because their body doesn't perform the way it used to.

Chiropractic is part of a healthy lifestyle. It's not the be all, do all, end all, but it is a significant piece of a healthy lifestyle. Every choice we make helps us become stronger and healthier or closer to dead and dying.

Question: How can someone find out more about Optimum Wellness Solutions?

Dr. Nannis: The easiest way is to give my office a call at 972-671-2225 and schedule a consultation. They can also go to our website www.optimumwellnesssolutions.com or our Facebook page: Optimum Wellness Solutions.

Come to any of our workshops. We have basic workshops every other week and advanced workshops at least once a month.

CHAPTER FOUR

Dr. Hong Yim

Horizon Wellness Center, Inc.

DR. HONG B. YIM

Dr. Hong B. Yim is a chiropractic physician with specialties in sports medicine and nutrition. He has extensive training in traditional Chinese medicine, a process which uses acupuncture and herbs, that he gained from his study abroad in Beijing, China. He is a certified Kinesio Taping instructor and provides education in the Kinesio Taping method to other chiropractors, physical therapists, occupational therapists, massage therapists, athletic trainers, and other health related practitioners.

Dr. Yim has lectured on various topics such as acupuncture, Kinesio Taping, nutrition, sports medicine, sports nutrition, and fitness. Dr. Yim has completed several marathons and ironman triathlons while active as an endurance athlete. He coaches and trains using functional training methodology, body weight exercises, and activities that enhance day-to-day activities.

Conversation with Dr. Yim:

Question: Please tell us about your practice and the patients you serve.

Dr. Yim: My interest is actually in performance enhancements. My current patients range from your typical neck and back chiropractic patients to patients with complex neuropathy, stomach problems, poor digestion, indigestion, acid reflux, heart conditions, cancer, weight management, and people looking to improve their general health. I do a lot with traditional Chinese medicine, using natural herbs, vitamins, and supplements to help improve health, wellness, and function.

Question: How do you help with neuropathy?

Dr. Yim: There are several different causes of neuropathy. Sometimes it's from pinched nerves of the spine, such as spinal stenosis. Other times, vascular or blood circulation issues compromise nerve function. In other cases, it's from an adverse reaction to chemo for cancer patients, which leads to neuropathy that lingers after treatments are completed. The body loses that control mechanism for normal nerve function, and you end up with either the sensation of numbness and tingling, or pain. I use acupuncture, typically, for that, and depending on the individual's age, I may use some supplements to help with their nervous system's general health as well as to combat the effects nerve irritation.

Question: What made you decide to become a chiropractor?

Dr. Yim: Chiropractic is an alternative compromise, halfway between a MD and a physical therapist. What I wanted was not to dispense medications like in the traditional medical realm, because most doctors, when you go see them, the MDs, they will actually write a script and you're pretty much done, and you leave the same way you entered. I wanted to provide something more than a PT who does a lot of the physical, rehabilitation activities. I wanted to be able to properly diagnose and have a little more say in the diagnostic component without actually prescribing drugs. Chiropractic is a wonderful and rewarding career. I thought that I could use my hands to heal, and as a doctor, I could diagnose their conditions and analyze them in a way that most PTs may, or may not, have the opportunity to do. It gave me the ability and power to be able to diagnose and treat using my hands, rather than with medicine.

Question: It sounds like you have a lot of background in naturopath information, too. Can you talk about that?

Dr. Yim: I've always had an interest in natural medicine. I have always felt that the body can heal itself. You look at the phenomenon of animals. There isn't extensive medicine for animals; they don't have health insurance in the way that we do. Instead, food is medicine because food can heal as well as kill. Naturopathic medicine allows for the idea that using certain types of supplements or herbs can help give the body a boost that will allow it to regain normal function.

Question: Can you share a lesson you learned early on that still impacts how you run your practice today?

Dr. Yim: I've been in practice over 20 years. I built a strong foundation for what I wanted and what I didn't in my own practice based on what I witnessed while filling in for other doctors as a graduate in chiropractic school. Some of the practices were run traditionally, where all they do is neck and back. Another one was a mill or factory where they saw a high volume of patients and didn't spend much time with each individual. One of the key things in my practice is my belief in developing a relationship with a patient, and taking the time to listen to what they have to say. Even in school, my professor used to say, "If you listen to the patient, 90% of the diagnosis will be found in the history, but you have to spend the time to actually listen." That's one of the things that I value in my practice that I take time with each of my patients to listen carefully, then make my diagnosis. Whenever they come in, I listen, and I ask questions. Not only about them, but about their family as well.

Learning about the patient gives me a good picture of what's going on in their lives. Studying Oriental medicine teaches me how the relationships of the patient to their significant other, spouses, relatives, or other family members, work environment, and their life outside influence the health and wellness of the individual.

Question: Can you break down, based off of your experience, how much of that is emotional versus physical?

Dr. Yim: Accidents are fairly easy; they are a straight cause and effect relationship. When you have more complex cases that develop gradually or at random, Oriental medicine has provided other means of explanations as to how certain problems or pains arise. Back pain in Oriental medicine, comes from weakness of the kidney. Not that you necessarily have a kidney problem, but the energy around the kidney resides in your lower back. When you cannot support the muscle structures and bones, it can lead to weaknesses of that entire support system, thus leading to the back pain.

Having said that, the kidney is where your life energy, or chi, is contained. Food and water is combined and converted from the stomach and then stored in the kidneys. Emotions are also connected to that. The stomach organ deals with worry and concern, the kidneys deal with fear. Fear can lead to kidney problems, or a weak lower back, thus leading to susceptibility of low back pain.

Question: Let's say you discover somebody who is living in fear. How do you help them get past that?

Dr. Yim: The first step is to develop awareness of what that fear is. My job is to present and demonstrate what I find from my analysis, or evaluation using pulse and tongue diagnosis, and other methods, and say, "here are some fear factors in your life that I think may be contributing to your specific issues." Then I would proceed to find out how that fear component injures or weakens them physically. Awareness is just the beginning of the healing phase. Action is the last and most difficult part. Without the awareness, you cannot make a change.

Question: How do you help them address the action?

Dr. Yim: This depends on the actual problem at hand. For example, I've had patients who have a history of abuse in the family, or some traumatic event in their life. Typically, those patients will already have a therapist. I perform pulse and tongue diagnosis using traditional Chinese medicine approaches. A pulse diagnosis is a technique from Oriental medicine used to determine what is going on in a particular individual. This helps me to look into their emotional and physical states. When I bring up what the pulse diagnosis indicates, the patient almost always shares part of their history that they haven't divulged. My goal is to understand the individual so that I can treat their condition better.

Question: What are some of the benefits of using a chiropractor?

Dr. Yim: Chiropractic has always been a concept of healing by hand, *chiros practicos*. Chiropractic, for most conditions of the neck and back, are great. Most chiropractors are trained to look at the individual as a whole, not just their symptoms. By doing so, each chiropractor is moved to care about the patient's general health and wellbeing, not just their current condition. Chiropractors tend to be more knowledgeable of natural medicine, and alternative approaches to treating various conditions. Most people go to chiropractors not only for their neck or back pain, but also for wellness. We, as chiropractors, always want to bring the body back to homeostasis so that it can heal itself with the right support.

Question: What are some myths and misconceptions people generally have about chiropractic?

Dr. Yim: Mostly that chiropractor are thought of as neck and back crackers. Yes, we do adjust the spine and it makes a noise. We try to dissuade patients from saying, "crack" because it sounds horrible. A lot of people have misconceptions that a chiropractor will hurt them. There are cases where that is true, and it's all on an individual basis. You go to a dentist or a doctor; they may make your teeth or condition worse, who knows? But in general, they're there to help you. Most chiropractors don't have a very busy, seeing a hundred patients a day practice and will spend time to educate their patients on all aspects of the procedures and treatments.

Chiropractors are probably one of the better educators in medicine at explaining to the patient what is happening to their body and how to take better care of themselves, rather than just writing a scrip or treating the symptoms.

Question: What fears do you find that people have of chiropractic?

Dr. Yim: The fears that arise with chiropractic for most patients are with the neck and the noise associated with manipulation or an adjustment. No one likes to have their neck twisted, or turned in funny ways. A lot of the bad press says that when you get your neck adjusted, you'll have a stroke. In school we're always taught that before you do a neck adjustment, you should assess the dangers and risks posed to the individual by performing a vertebral artery screen. This identifies certain patients who may or may not be at risk for problems associated with a neck adjustment. Having said that, not all neck adjustments are the same. We use different techniques to ensure minimal risk to the patient. We have instruments to assist in the adjusting to avoid problems or concerns for patients who are tentative about having the traditional manipulation to the neck. The statistics say you're not really at that much of a risk.

The vertebral artery has been dissected in some cases, but those patients had other risk factors, which should have been taken into account prior to adjusting. It is unfortunate that things happen, but over three hundred thousand people die as a result of medical negligence in hospitals, and no one really complains too much about that, right? Accidents happen and everyone tries to do what's best for the patient and sometimes, even the best-laid plans are destined to fail. Despite the fact that most of the manipulation and strokes associated were not done by chiropractors, since we manipulate the spine /neck, we get the blame.

Question: It's interesting that chiropractors get the blame.

Dr. Yim: Of course, because we're the ones who manipulate. Some PTs manipulate, which is not necessarily legal, but there is a fine line between mobilization and manipulation. I've seen massage therapists doing manipulations, too. We are specifically trained for performing manipulation and other professions are not, that's the bottom line.

Question: That's scary.

Dr. Yim: It is, because their training is very different. There is always potential for something to go wrong even with the best training. Think of the surgeries that go awry. We need to be wary of everything we do, regardless of training or experience.

Question: How have you been able to help patients overcome obstacles? Can you describe a situation where you helped a patient feel better by overcoming a misconception or fear?

Dr. Yim: Lot of times. When I have a patient who is hesitant or resistant, I educate them. Being a chiropractor/doctor is part being a teacher as well. Just because a teacher says certain things, you don't have to follow their advice. My job as a teacher, instructor, doctor, and physician is to provide the information to allow the patient to make their own educated and informed decision about what needs to be done. Educating the patient lays the foundations for the validity of what I'm trying to do. In this way, the patient understands from the beginning to the end what the plan is, how we expect to proceed, and the outcome(s) we expect.

In some cases, I will also provide the possible negative outcomes. Look, we have the best-laid plan. Even though we are being careful, here's what could happen. If you are willing to follow my recommendations after that, then you can proceed with your current therapy. If not, when you're ready, please come back and we can work together. I don't like to push patients to choose, but I give them the option and opportunity to question and make informed decisions about their care. The patient should always be given the opportunity to weigh their options and make whichever choice is best for them.

Question: Have you ever had patients who were scared, but when you educated them, their fear suddenly evaporated?

Dr. Yim: Yes, because I give them the all the fact and statistics. Their fear is usually present because they're unfamiliar with the process. When I explain the entire process, what I am going to do, the goals we will try to achieve, and why they're having issues, the fears fade away. Let's say, for example, we're going to adjust the neck. The sound you hear is gasses within the joints. Imagine if you had rows of bubble wrap, and at some point there was a wrinkle. You put something heavy down on it and you hear a pop, right? Then it sort of levels out.

Well, your joints are the same way. The gasses within your joints are under asymmetrical pressure, so when we adjust, we release those gasses to realign the spine and keep you more balanced. You may or may not hear a pop when the gasses leave and then redistribute to level out your spine. That is part of the alignment process. Will you have pain? Not necessarily, but you are going to look for improved function before pain may be alleviated. Depending on the duration of pain, we always look for objective and measurable changes before subjective changes are noted.

Question: What's the one thing that we haven't covered that you would like to share with someone who is considering chiropractic?

Dr. Yim: I think the individual should have an open mind or desire to seek an alternative approach to their health problems. Always get a recommendation or referral if you're not sure who to go to. Tell them everything. Make sure you understand, and you're given a full explanation of where your condition stems from, the cause as well as the results, and the process by which you are going to become better. A complete treatment plan should be outlined on the first visit or shortly there afterwards.

Question: How can someone find more information about your practice?

Dr. Yim: I have a website: www.horizonwellnessskokie.com. They can also look me up on kinesiotaping.com; I am a CKTI, or certified KinesioTaping instructor. This is the taping technique used by the Olympic athletes, but the majority of the uses are in the non-athletic population.

CHAPTER FIVE

Dr. Dan Lavanga

Lavanga Holistic Center

Dr. Dan Lavanga

Dr. Dan Lavanga graduated from Sherman Chiropractic College in Spartanburg, South Carolina in 1986. He has practiced in Southampton, Pennsylvania since 1987 and studied extensively in multiple natural health sciences and techniques. Hischiropractic team focuses on family practice and specializes in low force advanced muscle therapy, sports, and extremity treatment as well as being highly skilled in various manual adjustment, mobilization, and manipulation techniques. Lavanga Chiropractic practitioners also utilize the "Arthrostimulator" a hand held device that delivers corrective adjustments without pain or manipulation.

Dr. Dan is known as the Doctor's Doctor. Many physicians come to him to get their health in alignment. His personal practice focuses on accomplished and highly stressed businessmen and women, and entrepreneurs. His practice includes chiropractic, nutrition, massage, life and business coaching, and consulting.

Conversation with Dr. Lavanga:

Question: Tell us about your practice and the patients you help.

Dr. Lavanga: I've been practicing in Southampton Pennsylvania since 1987. This is our 29th year. We are, I would say, a broad based practice. We see patients starting from infants, as well as athletes, marathon runners, etc. About 10% of my practice is motor vehicle accidents or work injuries. The majority of what we do is regular chiropractic cases. We're goal oriented. When people come in, we want to know what their goals are, and what they are looking to accomplish. They're looking for a good doctor and we're looking for a good patient.

When they come in, we introduce them to the practice with a video called "The Circle of Wellness". It basically tells them about the six facets of the work that we do: chiropractic, massage physiotherapy, exercise rehabilitation, detoxification, nutrition, and weight management. Then we add in our mental/emotional suggestions because we know that stress is a big factor. We have a stress management program, and we also do some coaching and personal development. We introduce them to the physical, chemical, and mental/emotional aspects of curative, natural, and holistic healthcare.

When they come in we do the doctor thing. We do a history, a thorough examination, find out everything we can about them, reports, whatever we need to do, and then we have them come back for a report of findings before we lay out a very individualized program including length of care, costs, etc. They may just need some chiropractic work or all seven facets of care for their physical, chemical, and emotional wellbeing.

We specialize in taking a cutting edge, holistic view of the patient. What we've found over the last ten to fifteen years is that we get much more compliance and much better results from folks by addressing all facets of their health and lifestyle, not just the pain part.

When I first started in practice, it was hardly anything more than adjustments of the spine. I thought I had miraculous lightning bolts in my hands and chiropractic could cure everybody. We found out as we went along that some people got well, and others didn't, so that's why we started to look at other aspects of their wellness.

Question: Why did you become a chiropractor?

Dr. Lavanga: I love that question because it's such a great memory for me. I started my career out of high school in a steel factory. My dad was a steel worker. I was in the United Auto Workers Union for 10 years. I became a machinist. I was terrific with machines. About six or seven years into that, I saw the future of that business; it was right around the time of the first gas crisis in this country. I saw the writing on the wall and figured that I probably wouldn't get 30 years in the auto industry, so I started to look for something else.

Physical therapy was big then, so I looked into becoming a physical therapist. By good fortune, a coworker introduced me to my first chiropractor, Dr. Mark Keminosh. I went to see Mark because I was interested in the career itself. He worked on me, worked with me, talked to me, and I realized that physical therapists worked for doctors and chiropractors were their own bosses.

After being in the steel factory and the union for ten years, I wanted to be my own boss. I decided chiropractic was for me, and for those selfish reasons, I found out about the philosophy behind chiropractic. It became inspirational for me to learn about the power of the human body, and how it worked. I love the mechanical parts of it. We use a lot of machines and tools in my office. I feel like I'm fixing parts, just like I did back in the early and late 70s in the steel factory.

Question: Can you share a lesson you learned early on that still impacts how you run your practice today?

Dr. Lavanga: In maybe my fourth year in practice, we had a patient, a young woman, who was being treated for asthma that found some relief through chiropractic. We don't promote that we cure asthma. With manipulation of the thoracic spine, some asthmatics find their condition improves. This young woman insisted that I take a look at her nephew who was four or five years old, and in a coma due to an accidental drowning. The child had terrible labored breathing and she wanted to know if I could help.

This is way out of my scope of practice. I told her that wasn't in my field of expertise, but she harped until I saw the child. I was reticent to do the work, but as I felt the child's spine, I said, listen, this is what I could do; I could do a very low velocity, gentle manipulation with an instrument, without cracking bones to his thoracic spine, the upper spine. This is the same thing I do for asthmatics. I said that I didn't know if it was going to help or not, but it certainly wouldn't hurt to try. We did a series of manipulations, around three.

Secretly, I hoped for a miracle. What happened was the labored breathing had gone back to what it was before. Whatever the reason for the labored breathing, with chiropractic, the problem cleared. The lesson I learned was that it is not always in my power. Sometimes it's the power of healing, the power of chiropractic, and the power of love. Healing is relative to the person. Some people will never heal from back surgery or from a divorce or loss, but if you can make them more comfortable and more viable, more vital, then you've done your job.

Question: What are some health benefits of using a chiropractor?

Dr. Lavanga: The mechanical aspect of chiropractic is beautiful. A spine has 24 movable bones that each interact with those above and below. The responsibility of those bones is to keep the communication system of the body (the nervous system) clear. Every spinal nerve goes where it's supposed to without being impinged or impaired or, as we like to say, subluxated or misaligned.

The first benefit of being under a chiropractor's care is that the mechanics of the spine are maintained. We can maintain those mechanics; I have patients in their 70s, 80s, and 90s who have been coming to me for years, and who are just as healthy now as they were in their 40s and 50s. They love the mechanics. Science tells us that when we manipulate a joint, we release endorphins, we release adrenalin, we release and free up blood flow, and nerve supply. This begins a healing process that may have been inhibited by this lack of nerve flow or blood supply to an area.

The second thing that occurs is that the chemistry of the body changes. When a person's physical body feels better, their chemistry becomes more balanced. When they have more balance in their life, they have a better outlook. I believe that some people come to me on a monthly basis simply because they want realignment. My motto is: when your spine is in line; you will feel fine.

We look at the well being of the entire person. Anything from the amount of stress they have in their life, to their diet, and physical activity, these can all benefit from having a thorough and well-tuned chiropractic alignment.

Question: What are some myths and misconceptions people have about chiropractic?

Dr. Lavanga: One of the main misconceptions people have is about how often you have to see a chiropractor. People always think you have to come back again and again. The truth is, I give recommendations, but I can't make people do something they don't want to. We have people that come in once a week for a lifetime. I don't make them come in; they come because they see some benefit in it.

Some people become addicted to the adjustments and I tell them that they need less care. I'll put them on a once a month or every other month plan; I'm not interested in over manipulating anybody. For the most part, people come because they see value in the service.

Another misconception is about the expense of what we do. People, for some reason, think that we're all driving Bentleys and living in Beverly Hills. We make a modest living doing a very important job that we work hard at, and we're basically less than 1% of the entire medical budget as a group of 40,000-60,000 chiropractors.

Perhaps the worst myth is that chiropractic adjustments can harm people. The best objective proof that this is a myth is that chiropractic treatment is rated as one of the safest medical treatments. Further proof can be found in data regarding our malpractice insurance rates. In my almost 30 years as a chiropractor, the rates are low and they continue to go down. In 1987, we paid $2500.00 per year in Pennsylvania and in 2016 we pay $1850.00. If insurance companies were paying out millions of dollars because of negligence in the chiropractic profession, our numbers would be through the roof. They wouldn't be the same or going down after 30 years.

Question: What are some common fears people have about chiropractic?

Dr. Lavanga: The cracking. Cracking that is going to break their neck. You know what, it's a valid fear. When someone puts their hands around your neck, especially for the first time, I don't blame people for being afraid, I know I was. Even though you're doing something good for them, sometimes the fear itself is worse than the benefit of the cure. We've developed other methods for folks like that. We turn to more gentle methods or use instruments to perform the adjustments. We use a lot of deep tissue work. I've been in practice for 29 years and I've had massage therapists with me for 28 of those.

Question: How have you been able to help your patients overcome those fears or misconceptions?

Dr. Lavanga: Many times people are afraid to have their neck adjusted. We'll do certain movements called myofascial release, which is basically working with the musculature, some traction of the neck, and use some instrumentation. Often times, what happens when you're doing those little maneuvers are that the joint will manipulate itself.

Other times, we'll do what I always do at the first visit, the lightest possible adjustment. I'll tell them, listen, you may go home and you may say I don't think he did anything. I'd rather have that then they go home and not come back because the adjustment hurt. We always err on the cautious side to gain their trust. When a neck adjustment, manipulation, or something has to be done that they're afraid of, we do it with care, and explain the entire process. Or we find an alternative method. I have a high referral rate for new patients because people trust my team and I. Those who trust me send people that trust them, and that's how trust is built over time. We're in a good place as far as that goes. That's how we overcome those typical fears.

Question: What is the one thing that we haven't covered that you would share with someone who is considering chiropractic?

Dr. Lavanga: We haven't spoken about different organic conditions people have that may actually be due to a nervous system issue. Going all the way back to colicky babies. It's funny; I remember a story about Donald Trump. Marla Maples and Donald Trump went to a chiropractor for a colicky child. It was a big story, probably in the National Enquirer back then since he had buddies working there. It was great for us because here you have a positive story of this celebrity who took their infant to a chiropractor for colic. Many people think, "What are you nuts, taking a baby to a chiropractor?"

That is one thing that people need to understand. If children are having issues like ear infections, colic, or things like that, we are not a cure, but sometimes an alignment will help to restore their health. If it's only 50% of the time, 10%, or even 1%, I still think it's worth the visit.

The other thing is a rampant overuse of medications for depression, anxiety, irritable bowel syndrome, and other conditions like that. These conditions sometimes stem from the body being out of balance or homeostasis, from poor dietary choices, and/or lack of exercise. At our center, we utilize the holistic approach of the Circle of Wellness System and often, with a few weeks of care, the body becomes more balanced. From that point, we look at what the patient is putting in their body. A lot of people don't even realize they're poisoning themselves. For some people, maybe 10%, a gluten free diet might be ideal, but it's not for everybody. It might be getting off of dairy, it might be getting off of wheat, or it might just be cutting out the everyday stress. We offer stress management programs, meditation, and yoga in our office. Sometimes people just need to be centered in their lives.

Question: How can someone find out more about your practice?

Dr. Lavanga: First, thank you for the opportunity to talk about chiropractic and holistic health. We are available almost everywhere. On the web: lavangachiropractic.com. We have an 888-LAVANGA number and our main number is 215-364-1112. You can Google Dr. Dan in Feasterville or Southampton, Pennsylvania. I have a lot of YouTube videos out there on personal training and stress management, as well as a number of books on the subjects.

CHAPTER SIX

Dr.Steven Buras

Jones Road Chiropractic

DR. STEVEN BURAS

Dr. Steven Buras specializes in the evaluation, treatment, and rehabilitation of the neck, back, and extremities. Dr. Buras has been practicing chiropractic since 1992. He earned his bachelor's degree from Texas A&M University and his doctorate in chiropractic from Texas Chiropractic College. He is a native of Houston. Dr. Buras has been married to his wife, Lisa, since 1993 and has two terrific children. Besides his family, his hobbies include fishing, golf, working out, and most outdoor recreation. Dr. Buras is a devout believer in God and keeps Him at the center of his work.

Dr. Buras was introduced to chiropractic as a patient at the age of 18 following a neck injury. During the course of his recovery, he discovered the value of a healthy spine and proper alignment. Over the course of his career, he has learned the greater importance of maintaining health through an active lifestyle and proper nutrition. He is committed to helping change the level of health in his patients and his community. He also enjoys fundraising for local charities, such as the Cypress Assistance Ministries, and the American Heart Association.

Conversation with Dr. Buras

Question: Please describe your practice and tell us about the patients you serve.

Dr. Buras: My practice is about 80 to 85 percent self-pay, group insurance patients. They are not motivated by financial gain for the most part. We do see a sprinkling of auto accidents as well. The patients I get most excited about are those who have no idea what chiropractic is. I take the greatest satisfaction out of treating migraine patients. They seem so debilitated by their headaches, and many have gone years that way. When you can help a patient attend loud social events or enjoy the sunlight in a way they haven't been able to for years, that's truly rewarding.

We also treat common neck and back complaints, and disc problems. Certainly we get satisfaction out of treating those as well. It's rewarding to get people active enough that they can enjoy their life again.

Question: Are migraine headaches a specialty for you?

Dr. Buras: I wouldn't say I specialize in them. I don't think any chiropractor could. I've been practicing for about 22, almost 23 years, and over that period of time you develop a certain expertise in one thing or another. I have pretty good success in treating them.

Question: Do migraine medicines continue to work over time or do they lose effectiveness?

Dr. Buras: There are certain drugs that are specific to migraines and they do their job. They all have their own side effects and they will suppress those headaches. The problem is that they still get the headaches, so they have to take those drugs either to prevent the headaches or treat them after the fact. I may be biased, but the better solution is to find the source of the problem and resolve it. Then you won't have to worry about the poison you put in your body to mask them.

Question: Is there an average time span it takes for you to help people with migraines?

Dr. Buras: I would say that it's usually a few weeks, maybe three or four, but it depends on the patient. One of the stories that stick out in my mind is of a 72 year old woman who had a history of migraines. The woman had two to three migraines a week for 50 years. She marked the start of her headaches from the end of World War II. Her sister had a similar history and was treated by a chiropractor. Hearing about her sister's success made her seek chiropractic care. After about two weeks, she stopped having migraines, but still had a low-grade headache all the time. It took about six weeks to relieve her of all headaches. She came back a year and half later and wanted to hug me because she still hadn't had a migraine. For her, it was nothing short of a miracle.

I've had other patients take a couple of months before they really begin to see results. Each patient is different, but I think on average, a migraine patient begins to see some relief in three weeks. It doesn't take very long.

Question: Do they typically have to go back for treatment?

Dr. Buras: Yes, it's a repetition in care because you have to ... Well, let me back up. Depending on the source of that headache, a lot of them are due to mechanical dysfunctions in the upper part of the neck. In order to get rid of the headaches, you can passively get rid of them with an adjustment or two, but you haven't changed the mechanical trigger that's causing them. You have to retrain function and movement back into those regions of the spine. It's like going to the gym to build muscle; you can't get stronger biceps if you only work out a couple times.

Repetition is key. Not only to feel better, but if you continue to work over a series of adjustments, then you can change the actual stimulator of the problem. It doesn't take six months for that to happen. It doesn't take a ton of time. It just takes repetition.

Question: What made you decide to be a chiropractor?

Dr. Buras: My own experience. I pinched a nerve in my neck when I was 18 years old. I couldn't turn my head, and it was the worst night's sleep I had ever had. My dad took me to the chiropractor that had treated my grandmother, and gotten rid of her migraine headaches. He adjusted me a couple of times, and I felt so much better after the first adjustment. That was my exposure to chiropractic. I wound up having a problem that took me a year to get corrected, and that second chiropractor really got me interested in the field.

Question: What about it interested you?

Dr. Buras: I thought it was a unique form of medicine. If you've been to a chiropractor, then you know it's not like going to your regular physician. It just interested me, the mechanics of it all. I guess the bio-mechanical aspects. I was weight lifting at the time, so it all seemed to fit together.

Question: What lesson did you learn early on that still impacts your practice today?

Dr. Buras: I have, over the last 10 years, or 12 years of my career, learned that you can truly impact somebody's health through chiropractic. Not just get rid of their pain. I treat my patients with the idea of significantly changing their future health. That mentality is a product of experience.

Question: Talk about the health benefits of using chiropractic.

Dr. Buras: People seek chiropractors because their neck or their back hurts, for the most part. That's probably what we are best known for. Our nervous system is housed inside our spine, and our spine is protection for our nervous system. When there's subluxation or dysfunction of the spine, it creates low-grade inflammation. That inflammation then affects the nerves around that region, and the inflammation of those nerves then affects the nerve's ability to do its job. A real simple example is that when somebody has low back pain, they will sometimes become constipated. This is because the nerves are not sending signals to the colon to do the job that it is supposed to. It has been well documented that adjustments can affect blood pressure, heart rate, allergies, and many other organ dysfunctions. It's a matter of relieving stress and inflammation from the spine.

Question: What are some myths and misconceptions that people have about chiropractic?

Dr. Buras: People are scared that they will have their neck broken during an adjustment. I'm sure it's happened somewhere, but I've never heard of it. It would take a really aggressive force to break somebody's neck, and I just don't know that you could do that with an adjustment. Well, I'll back that up, and say that older physicians are of the opinion that chiropractors actually damage discs and your spine. The noise that you hear when you get an adjustment is nothing more than gas bubbles forming in the joints of the spine. The same as when you crack your knuckles on your hands. The misconception is that when you hear that loud pop, that something is being destroyed or damaged. The misconception is that chiropractic is dangerous to the spine, and the reality is, that it is not.

Question: Are there any controversial topics in chiropractic that people talk about?

Dr. Buras: Some chiropractors are of the opinion that there's no need for outside medicine whatsoever, that chiropractic cures everything. I think there's some discussion to be had there. On the other hand, I really think that chiropractic has its place alongside traditional medicine as well.

There's some discussion that you could kill somebody with a stroke to the neck, and frankly, that's absolutely true. A responsible chiropractor, though, is going to screen a patient for that. In a certain population, you don't want to do an upper cervical adjustment because there is a risk of stroke for the patient. It's pretty minor. In fact, it's almost rare.

Question: What are some common fears that people have about chiropractic?

Dr. Buras: There's an old criticism that if you go to chiropractor, you have to go a hundred times, and you'll get addicted. There's no addiction to chiropractic, and it doesn't create a dependence on chiropractic either. The reason people come back for maintenance care for a lifetime is that they realize they're healthier when they do. That's the bottom line. Getting adjusted doesn't create a dependency on chiropractic. It's the same as exercise. You're not addicted to exercise either, but it's healthy to do it and makes you feel good.

Question: Do people fear chiropractors?

Dr. Buras: They certainly do; for the reasons we already talked about. Breaking your neck, or damaging a disc, and that kind of thing. Honestly, that's propagated, too, by some of the physicians in the medical community.

Question: How have you been able to help patients overcome their obstacles?

Dr. Buras: Well, we try hard to educate our patients. When I see a patient for the first time, I rarely, if ever, adjust them that day. We go through an education process so that the patient is comfortable with what we're doing. I think when you eliminate the patient's fear, and prepare them for that loud noise when they get adjusted; they are much better equipped to handle that first time anxiety. Once they realize that you're not going to injure them, they are much more comfortable.

That's the second thing that they need to get over, their fear that it's going to hurt to get adjusted. When you have a patient that comes in and they're in pain already, they believe it's going to hurt. You have to educate the patient on what it is we do, why we do it, and what the health benefits are long term.

Question: What's the one thing that we haven't covered that you'd like to share with someone who is considering chiropractic?

Dr. Buras: I would tell you that, and I hate to sound like a billboard, but almost everybody needs chiropractic. The American way is to eat too much, exercise too little, and to work long hours at a desk. Those three things tend to conspire together to destroy our health. Most of our health conditions area self-inflicted. Our poor diet, in America, has led to obesity being higher than it's ever been, and again our lifestyle is one that's very sedentary. We never walk anywhere. We have a car to take us where we want to go, and we sit at our desk all day, we come home, we sit on the couch, and watch TV until we go to bed, and do it again the next day. Our bodies become overweight, deconditioned, and those two factors are probably, believe it or not, what lead to more back problems than any industrial accident ever could.

The patient population is ever expanding. The younger generation has grown up with a smart phone in their hand, and their neck is tipped forward all day from reading texts, and surfing the web. The coming years are going to have an epidemic of neck problems because of that.

Question: How can someone find out more about Jones Road Chiro?

Dr. Buras: Visit my website at www.jonesrdchiro.com. That is probably the best way to find us, find out what we do, what we believe, and how we treat. The phone number is 281-807-9210 or you can email us at drbures@jonesrdchiro.com. We also have a Facebook page: Jones Road Chiro.

CHAPTER SEVEN

Dr. Phillip Reyes

Clinton Chiropractic

DR. PHILLIP REYES

Dr. Phillip Reyes is a licensed chiropractor serving the Alameda community.

Dr. Phillip Reyes has been freeing people from pain in the clinic in Alameda, CA. As a chiropractor with experience, Dr. Reyes is committed to promoting optimal health and wellbeing of patients.

Dr. Reyes uses a "whole person approach". This approach to wellness means looking for underlying causes of any disturbance or disruption (which may or may not be causing symptoms at the time) and recommending whatever interventions and lifestyle adjustments to optimize the conditions for normal function. Using this unique approach, Dr. Reyes is able to help you accelerate and/or maintain your journey to good health.

Our practice specializes in treating a variety of conditions, from chronic low back and neck pain to acute injuries caused by an accident or injury. Dr. Reyes is also a certified chiropractic sports physician, certified Industrial Disability Examiner and inventor of the Suportapedic back support (a unique, patent pending full spine and neck support Dr. Reyes designed for use on exercise equipment). Dr. Reyes is also one of a few centers locally (at the time of this entry) using the latest technology for soft tissue and sports injuries. The technology is called low level laser therapy or cold laser therapy. Dr. Reyes works at one of a few centers that used the cold laser in clinical trials. Recently, the FDA approved the low level laser for use on patients with carpal tunnel syndrome. This has proven to reduce symptoms, thereby decreasing the need for surgery.

Conversation with Dr. Reyes:

Question: Tell me about your practice and the patients you serve.

Dr. Reyes: Well, I've been practicing since 1988, so I've seen quite a few patients. I'm a certified chiropractic sports physician. The patients that I enjoy taking care of most are the run of the mill back pain patients that have gone through the medical field and have not gotten any help. It's your basic chiropractic cases that keep me in business. What's been rewarding is seeing people who have had a significant amount of back pain that limited what they could do, and being able to help them enjoy those activities again. I've kind of gone the full gamut. I've seen some difficult cases, even the worst surgical cases.

Question: Is there something that you specialize in?

Dr. Reyes: No, I do a lot of different things and I think that's what keeps the practice interesting. I see sports injuries, personal injury cases, and back pain patients. I've got seniors and I've got young people. That kind of variety keeps things lively around here.

Question: What difference are the outcomes making in their lives?

Dr. Reyes: I had one guy who took forever to come in. His wife was a current patient. He had severe low back pain; he couldn't even get out of bed in the morning. He was very reluctant to get chiropractic care because he'd been to medical doctors and orthopedics in the past and he was more inclined to utilize medical care; however, the medical care was not helping with his condition.

He used to love playing golf and hadn't played for many years due to pain. When he finally came in, we did an examination and x-rays. I thought I could help him. He already had some significant degenerative changes in his lower back. When I went over the findings, he decided he didn't want to pursue any treatment, even though he was here twice already. It took him a year to come back and during that year he was still in a severe pain, but he took a chance and after one treatment, he felt significantly better.

He turned out being one of my best patients. He was able to go out and book weekend golf trips with his buddies that he hadn't been able to for a long time. Now he plays golf for two or three days, sometimes two rounds a day. So something like that, where somebody thought they wouldn't be able to do something they love and we were able to help them. It's pretty rewarding to see something like that.

Question: What made you decide to become a chiropractor?

Dr. Reyes: I've always been interested in health care. When I was a little kid, I found myself running towards kids that where hurt; whenever someone fell down and scraped their knees, I was the kid running to help when others ran away. I didn't know I wanted to be a chiropractor as a kid, but I knew I wanted to help people. I was fascinated by what the human body was capable of, if you took care of it, exercised, and ate well. I was also fascinated by the phenomenal accomplishments the body could achieve it is pushed it to its limit.

A negative experience with medication steered me away from the medical field. Although I had some issues with allergies and asthma that the medication helped me with, I had horrible side effects. I wanted to find an alternative to medicine that could prevent/and or treat injuries, illnesses, and pain in a natural way, without the negative side effects that medicine could have. The more I learned about chiropractic, the more it made sense, especially with respect to evaluating and treating sports injuries. Chiropractic can prevent problems that people had to take medication for in the first place.

Question: What is something one of your patients would consider miraculous that you helped them with?

Dr. Reyes: Well, let's see. One of the ladies that just left is in her 80s and back and forth to a medical doctor. She's on a lot of different medications, but doesn't like taking them. She is on gabapentin, morphine, and other medications that create other problems that she is trying to limit. She's been going to chiropractors her entire adult life, and is still an RN in her 80s. Thirty or 40 years ago when she first started going to chiropractors it was kind of taboo. A lot of nurses were going to chiropractors even though the medical doctors, at the time, were saying not to. Going to a chiropractor enabled her to get around pain free.

Question: Can you share a lesson that you learned early on that still impacts how you run your practice?

Dr. Reyes: When I first graduated from chiropractic school, I worked with a doctor in San Francisco. I was very impressed with how organized he kept everything. The organizational aspect of his office was something I wanted to replicate. He had a very smooth running office. He had a high volume practice seeing 60 patients or 70 patients a day, and it was very well run. He had a good staff, good flow, and good procedures from the front office to the back office to marketing. There are so many aspects to a practice to keep it going, to keep it productive, and to keep it in the positive. I think you have to have a good plan, good organization, and stay on top of everything. That impressed me most, and is probably what set me straight and has allowed me to be in practice for 28 years.

Question: What are some of the health benefits of using a chiropractor?

Dr. Reyes: It's difficult to attract people that are younger and get them to understand the benefits of chiropractic care. As we get a little older, we start to grasp what our limitations are, and how staying healthy as we age is really important. I think the hardest thing for me is to persuade the younger people to come in, and to instill in them the importance of maintaining things when they're younger. They may not be in pain, but some of the symptoms are still there; decreased ranges of motion, stiffness, aches, and so forth after activities. If we get them in and educate them when they are younger, it will be better for them down the road.

One health condition in particular that I have witnessed first-hand is that chiropractic adjustments help with heartburn. If I have not had an adjustment in a while, I will develop ongoing heartburn that returns as soon as the OTC medication wears off. Within minutes of getting an adjustment, the heartburn ceases. A certain percentage of people with chronic heartburn can also develop Barretts' Esophagus, which is a condition that can become cancerous. So for me, it may be helpful in warding off this condition, and it certainly helps me with my heartburn. The literature states that about 60 million Americans suffer from heartburn at least once per month. Think of how many people that could benefit from a natural treatment for this condition.

Question: There are many fears and misconceptions in the chiropractic field. What are some that you have seen?

Dr. Reyes: It's always interesting to talk to people about why they don't go to a chiropractor. The answers are pretty varied. From things as basic as it sounds like it hurts. That is often not the case. Sometimes when people are in a lot pain, everything is a little uncomfortable. Generally, when people are in a lot of pain, their range of motion is limited, and I may not do a full on manipulation. There are a lot of things that we can do to make them to feel better, so that when we finally do an adjustment it's comfortable.

I think another myth is that people fear after you get started that you have to go forever. People think of health care practitioners like a one and done situation, where you go in, get a treatment, and you're done; you'll never have to go back.

You don't have to continue to go to chiropractic doctors, but I think that once people feel the benefits, they want to go. Some people fear starting because they think that they're going to have to go for the rest of their life in order to feel normal. Some people that have never been don't want to start because of that misconception.

Question: What are some more common fears that you've heard?

Dr. Reyes: Well, there's always the financial aspect. Some people don't have health care benefits, so there's always a concern with the cost of care. You can't really put a price on health and if you don't have good health, you can't continue to work, and you can't continue to enjoy your life. The cost factor is based on value. If they understand that it is going to allow them to continue doing the things that they enjoy in life, then it makes a lot of sense to them.

Question: Can you describe a situation where you helped a patient overcome a misconception or fear and helped them feel better?

Dr. Reyes: I think educating them is key. I had somebody yesterday that was talking to another person about coming in and the other person joked that once you start seeing a chiropractor, you have to go forever. I told her it's like going to a dentist. When you go to a dentist, nobody thinks twice about continuing. You use your body all the time. When you go to a dentist, you understand that you use your teeth every day. It's the same with chiropractic care. Educating the patient that they don't have to continue to see chiropractic often, but that there are benefits if they do, really helps put it in perspective.

Question: What's the one thing we haven't covered that you want to share with someone who is considering chiropractic?

Dr. Reyes: I guess that chiropractic is something people should incorporate as part of their normal healthy lifestyle. If someone is interested in maintaining their health, they need to take responsibility for their own health. Those are the people that seem to get the most out of chiropractic care, the best out of their health, and are able to continue to do things that they enjoy. Without our health, we really don't have much.

Question: How can someone find out more about your practice?

Dr. Reyes: They can always call and schedule a consultation. We do have a website so they can get more information there. The website is alamedachiropractor.com. Our website is fairly interactive. They can post a question and I'll get back to them. They can always call us at our phone number 510-865-1355. Schedule a consultation. We do a free consultation, and talk to patient to see if there's something that chiropractic care can help them with. If not, we have a list of doctors that we can refer them to. They can also email us at phillipreyesdc@gmail.com.

CHAPTER EIGHT

Dr. Bradley Mouroux

Mouroux Chiropractic

DR. BRADLEY MOUROUX

About Dr. Mouroux:

Dr. Bradley Mouroux is a native of California; born in Morgan Hill, he has lived in the South Valley for over 30 years. He graduated U.C. Davis with a B.S. degree in Cellular biology. Dr. Mouroux went on to perform stem cell research as a biologist and achieved accolades from his peers. It was later in his career that his own health problems led him to seek chiropractic care and as a result, changed his life and career forever. His overwhelmingly positive results inspired him to become a doctor of chiropractic and a leader of health and wellness in both his family and community. Dr. Mouroux continuously hones his skills by staying on top of current health news and educating his patients on the latest in health care. His focus is to help children and adults alike, achieve fantastic health through lifelong chiropractic care. As a health professional, he is a board certified chiropractor, professional applied kinesiologist, and a chiropractic sports physician. His expertise is in pediatric care, sports injury, automotive injury, neurologic disorders, allergy testing, and nutritional counseling/testing.

Conversation with Dr. Mouroux:

Question: Tell us about your practice and the patients you serve.

Dr. Mouroux: My practice is a chiropractic clinic that focuses on holistic whole body health. It also involves some of the core principles of chiropractic: neuromuscular balance, biomechanical balance, and nutritional consultation. We focus on all three aspects when working with our patients. We try not to overwhelm them with everything that we do all at once. We initially cater to what they need. If we find that they need more, we help them through the process of getting back their health, and their desired lifestyle.

Question: Let's talk about the outcomes you help achieve.

Dr. Mouroux: Generally speaking, we help people with low back pain, and neck pain, mainly from automobile accidents, people working too long with computers, sports, and work related injuries. We also get people who come in as a last resort or they've been everywhere else, and don't know where else to turn. Those are people that have migraine headaches, vertigo, or dizziness. Normally, they'll have some level of chronic inflammation and pain from poor diet, repetitive stress, and poor spinal maintenance. They'll have problems with neuropathic symptoms from diabetes. They'll have... gosh; it comes down to all different types of things. You'll have combinations of problems from someone that has low back pain, but also has issues with insomnia, carpal tunnel syndrome, arthritis, and disc bulge or disc herniation, fatigue, chronic fatigue, fibromyalgia, or temperomandibular joint problems. They might have all combinations of these things at once, and we focus on treating them all simultaneously. A lot of times, disease processes actually build and interfere with the normal workings of the body creating more body dysfunction.

For example, diabetes starts off just as diabetes, but can instigate muscle and joint problems, nerve problems, heart problems, eye and vision problems; they all stem from the diabetes. If we don't address the core issue of diabetes, as well as the other symptoms, then we're fighting a losing battle.

Question: Do you specialize in something in particular?

Dr. Mouroux: I guess what I specialize in is a method of analysis. I practice what's called professional applied kinesiology, which is an in depth study of body movement, and muscle function as it relates to organ system function. I use this in the majority of my patient cases to help get through sticking points or unresolved issues. I also have a specialization in ergonomics, and chiropractic sports medicine.

Question: What made you decide to become a chiropractor?

Dr. Mouroux: I definitely did not decide to become a chiropractor early on. I never knew what chiropractor was until I was about 21 years old. At that point in time, I had been up at UC Davis, and part of the rowing team. I was a novice rower. It was through the 1996 to 1997 school year that I rowed for UC Davis, and by the end of that year, I came out with a chronic left knee bursitis, low back, and groin pain from the constant workouts on the water. Additionally, I had developed insomnia. I saw a chiropractor that summer, and it reduced the lower back and the knee pain, but the insomnia hadn't been helped. I continued on, and completed UC Davis with a degree in cellular biology. After that, I conducted some research and production work with stem cells.

I was in the industry for five years, still battling this insomnia that had come up from the 1996 to 1997 growing season. I couldn't figure out why I couldn't get a solid night's sleep. Until I finally said, you know what? I'm going to look for a holistic answer. In 2002, I found a holistic chiropractor in San Jose. I was about 25 at the time. I went to see this chiropractor over the next year. Within the first month, I went from only sleeping an average of about four to five hours a night to about six hours a night, which to an insomniac, is a huge difference.

I continued to get better. I hadn't realized what I lost. I stopped fearing sleep the more hours I was able to rest. I realized that the work I had been doing with stem cell research was only taking care of stroke patient damage, like brain damage after the fact. I wanted to focus more on the preventative end. I wanted to see how I could prevent myself from following a similar path of degenerative health. My results from chiropractic care opened my eyes to a new perspective. In that 2002 to 2003 time frame, I looked into become a chiropractor, but it wasn't until about 2007 that I finally got the guts to do it.

Once I got into the chiropractic college, and understood what chiropractic was about: balancing the nervous system, restoring balance through the body, healthier life choices, diet and correction of subluxation through the adjustment of the spine, I was hooked. This spoke volumes when it came to understanding what a true healthy lifestyle, and preventative healthcare was. That's where I felt like I had taken a step in the right direction. It is not a popular direction because chiropractic is misunderstood. Not everything you do is going to be popular.

Question: Can you share a lesson you learned early on that still impacts how you run your practice today?

Dr. Mouroux: That's a really good question. I think the lesson I learned earliest is that without a balanced lifestyle, health will always be lacking or unattainable. In my own right, I had to learn how to take care of myself, to take time to allow myself to sleep, allow myself to heal, allow myself to focus on how I ate, and on my lifestyle as a whole. If you don't focus on the things that you do every day, it doesn't matter what healthcare system you're in, whether or not you're doing chiropractic, whether or not you're taking medications through western medicine or acupuncture. If you don't focus on what you're doing on a daily basis to help maintain yourself, then you are destined to succumb to whatever happens. You're leaving yourself vulnerable. Our choices in life determine whether or not we will be healthy.

Question: There are plenty of health benefits to using a chiropractor. Can you talk about that?

Dr. Mouroux: I guess the biggest problem is that with chiropractic, you're not working on a particular condition, and in our society, we are condition based. The story goes kind of like this: "My neck hurts and I know where it is, but I'm not sure why it hurts and it does not seem to be getting better even when I work out and rest, can you fix it?" In chiropractic, the focus is to help balance the overall body by balancing out the nervous system function. The body is more complex than our linear thought process. It's not a simple one plus one equals two kind of thing.

It's really hard to tell somebody that yes, in two visits you're going to have no more neck pain because I know exactly what's happening. In chiropractic, it's more that we know when we help balance the spine; we help to normalize your nervous system function. After that, your body will continue to heal and balance itself out. The pain or the symptoms will eventually subside, reduce, or go away, but your health will be restored. The tough thing about chiropractic is that we're working on the bodies overall health and balance, which doesn't necessarily correlate to a particular condition or symptom. You do an adjustment, and it definitely relieves neck pain. You can say yes, that misalignment was causing that problem, but it's more of the latter, more that this adjustment helps the overall body, and structure balance. Over time, and with consistent work, just like working out, your body will become healthier and your symptoms will get better because you are functioning better.

It's like when you start working out, you don't get toned and strong overnight. You get strong as your body builds its stability and structure, as you condition yourself. You have to work at that. People say, why do I have to continue having chiropractic? Why do you have to continue brushing your teeth? Why do you have to continue working out? In order to make sure that anything is maintained in optimal condition, you have to work to maintain it. There's a certain amount of chiropractic that should be done on a regular basis. You can ask every chiropractor there is how often they get adjusted, and I'm willing to bet it would be at a minimum of once every two weeks. That's just to maintain their optimal nervous system balance, and function.

Question: What are some myths and misconceptions that people have about chiropractic?

Dr. Mouroux: I think the biggest myth is that there is no science behind it. Truth be told, chiropractic doesn't have a large research center affiliated with it because chiropractic is mainly made up of universities and sole practitioners working out of individual offices. Chiropractors don't have hospitals with chiropractic (which is a shame) or research centers of chiropractic. However, there's a lot of research being done by physical therapists, spine and disc specialists, and even MDs. Medical research has demonstrated that chiropractic spinal adjustments (called manipulations in the research) have many benefits, not only proving we do affect the nervous system function and the physiology of the body, but that chiropractic has positive effects on general health. Conditions such as arthritis, degenerative disc disease, and even problems of the body, like immune function, are all improved with chiropractic care. I'd say disease processes like Parkinson's, migraine headaches, asthma, high blood pressure, allergies, fatigue, cold, and immune function, all have positive responses with chiropractic care.

The second biggest misconception is that we're not actually doctors. The opposite is true. We are taught anatomy and physiology more than MDs. We know more about nutrition than medical doctors and we are taught more about neurology and physiology. We are a great first line of defense when it comes to pre-participation sports physicals, evaluating children, mothers before birth, and children after birth.

Birthing can be a traumatic process, and a lot of that can have effects on the baby and the mother. For example, issues with the baby's neck and spine can have profound effects on children when they start to develop. Things like croup, movement disorders, sleep, bowel, or digestive disorders, and asthma, can come about from a difficult birth.

Sometimes normal birth can be little harsh on a child's spine. When we think about what their first introduction was to the world, it was pretty darn rough. Getting them checked out is something that chiropractors do, and can do all the time. It's just not done enough.

Question: What are some common fears people have about chiropractic?

Dr. Mouroux: The number one fear is of having their neck hurt. Everyone that I've talked to fears getting their neck twisted off. It's funny because I had the same sort of fears before going to a chiropractor. In actuality, when I went through Chiropractic College, the opposite is true. It is to this date, to my knowledge, still recorded as being the safest medical procedure or non-medical procedure, depending on how you define it. We have the least costly malpractice insurance of almost any medical profession. Again, I don't have the numbers, but that's what we're told from the insurance professionals.

We spend very little on insurance when it comes to malpractice. Now can people feel pain after an adjustment? It's definitely possible. A lot of people come to us in a very unstable and delicate state, and sometimes there's no way to really know how unstable somebody is until we see how they respond after an adjustment. After the adjustment, if the client did have some pain, the biggest problem is having the patient understand that this is part of the process and if you stick with it a little longer, the most likely outcome is that the problem will continue to improve. Unfortunately, the fear of that pain is very real, but it's the same pain that is actually creating the spinal instability that they came in with in the first place.

They need to give it more time. It's kind of like any procedure. Sometimes things might not go well, but if you stick with it, it will continue to improve. Most people don't stick with it long enough; they get scared because they have all these fears of permanent damage. This is possible with any procedure, but extremely rare in chiropractic.

Question: What's the one thing we haven't covered that you would like to share with someone who is considering chiropractic?

Dr. Mouroux: There are many different styles of chiropractic. There are over 200 different techniques, specialties, and emphases that can be addressed through chiropractic. From neurology to nutrition to energy balancing, and energy/meridian work, the number one thing is that all chiropractors are different. When you find a chiropractor that works for you, like any doctor, don't let them go because you won't find another quite the same.

That's something I would say has not been talked about enough, the variability in our specialty. As professionals, we know that there are people that are chiropractic neurologists, chiropractic nutritionists, and even chiropractic sports medicine doctors, but it all depends on what their post-graduate education was.

Question: How can someone find out more about your unique take on chiropractic?

Dr. Mouroux: The best thing to do is go directly to the websites, or call for a free consultation. Secondly, take a look at reviews online. The people that review chiropractic will tell you volumes. They can be found on Yelp, Google reviews, or even by word of mouth.

You can find out more at my website, www.mourouxchirosanjose.com or visit me in person at Saratoga Rotary. Call our number 408-379-8888 and ask for a free consultation. My Facebook page is: Mouroux Chiropractic. Email us at:drmouroux@mourouxchirosanjose.com.

CHAPTER NINE

Dr. Doreen Lewis

DR. DOREEN LEWIS

Dr. Lewis has been practicing chiropractic in the San Antonio area for 28 years. She is a graduate of Texas Chiropractic College, class of 1984. Her style of practice is a blend of many techniques, including diversified, applied kinesiology, contact reflex analysis, total body modification, activator, nasal specific and acupuncture. She has also studied Brimhall, Thompson, Cox, Leander, SOT (Sacral Occipital Technique), HOI (Palmer, hole-in-one), Logan Basic, reflexology, and clinical kinesiology.

Dr. Lewis is board certified as a diplomat of the American Board of Chiropractic Internists and diplomat of the American Clinical Board of Nutrition. She is a certified clinical nutritionist, senior disability analyst and diplomat, and a Fellow of the International Academy of Medical Acupuncture. She has past experience as a certified laboratory technician from BAMC/Baylor University. Dr. Lewis is a certified naturopathic physician by the American Naturopathic Medical Certification Board. She is also an advanced graduate of the Spine Research Institute of San Diego.

Dr. Lewis is a member of the American Chiropractic Association, the Texas Chiropractic Association, the Texas State Naturopathic Medial Association, the Christian

Chiropractic Association, the American Academy of Chiropractic Physicians, the Medical Training Institute of America, the ACA Council on Nutrition, the International & American Association of Clinical Nutritionists, the ACA Council of Family Practice, and the TCC Alumni Association. She is also a lifetime member of Kingston's Who's Who and a past member of Who's Who of Executives and Professionals, for seven years.

Conversation with Dr. Lewis:

Question: Please describe your practice and the patients you serve.

Dr. Lewis: My practice is a little unusual. I have a double-edged clinic. One is called San Pedro North Chiropractic, and the other is Alpha Alternative Care Center. I have a lot of patients that just want chiropractic; I have a lot of patients who just want nutrition. I try to balance both, but it makes it quite challenging and very interesting. I've been practicing for 31 years. My favorite patient is the patient from 45 to 70 that is having problems with lupus or diabetes or change of life and hormones. Those types of patients are not part of the typical back practice that most chiropractors have.

As for an ailment like lupus, I'm not an MD. You have to understand what old-fashioned chiropractic was. Most chiropractors don't get it. Old-fashioned chiropractic treated the whole body. It's one unit, and when you get into lupus, you're getting into autoimmune diseases.

Autoimmune is a double-edged sword. You need two major traumas to trigger it. It can be a whiplash, it can be a divorce. It can be a fall down the stairs, it can be dietary. What we find with autoimmune diseases is that patients who get into type III sensitivities have 20 or more catatoxic allergies, more commonly known as food sensitivities. They have autoimmune kidney problems, or they have lung problems, which corresponds in Chinese medicine with the colon. When you look at this, you change their diets, and you get them on the right supplementations so that the antibodies in lupus start attacking the nutritional supplements. If you use a standard process product, you adjust the T12 for their kidneys. You check their lung function. We do spirometry and lung functions in the office. You check their lungs to make sure they don't have asthma, because usually if they have 20 or more allergies, they've got asthma.

It gets quite intensive, but you can bring people out of this pretty easy. There are some blood types you can't. Since I've been through it myself, I know how to do it.

Question: What made you decide to become a chiropractor?

Dr. Lewis: God told me this when I was 12, or 13 years old. I remember looking out the window-and I wasn't even a Christian at that time-when God spoke to me and told me I was going to be a chiropractor. I remember looking north at this beautiful world outside. I just knew at that moment that's what I was called to do. I've been passionate about it ever since.

Question: Did you know what a chiropractor was at that time?

Dr. Lewis: Yes, my mom had been in a car accident when I was a little girl and she was bedridden for my first two years of school. The doctors kept telling her to wear something warm around her neck and that they couldn't do anything else for her. She went to a DO the next town over in Massachusetts and the doctor of osteopathic medicine adjusted her. She was well in two months. My mom started taking us to chiropractors when she found out that chiropractors were better adjusters than osteopaths. Growing up, every two weeks we'd cross the state line to New Hampshire where we would get adjusted by an old-fashioned Palmer technique called the hole in one. Our atlas was adjusted every two weeks.

When chiropractic became legal in Massachusetts, it was a whole different story. We started seeing a female chiropractor in Worcester and she did my very first pap smear. It was very holistic. My mom started seeing another chiropractor in Lancaster to get her liver detoxed. I always grew up thinking chiropractors were a completely holistic practice. That's what I've tried to do, to be a holistic doctor. Now it seems like everything that chiropractors do, the MDs want to copy. We've been doing a lot of strange things in that office for a long time. Like the balloon sinuplasty technique that is all the rage right now. Chiropractors invented that technique in the 1930s. I've been doing it in the office now for 15 years.

They've come out with this brand new technique. They went to our courses and learned from us. It's very frustrating for me as a chiropractor to watch them take the reins on all things that we've been using for years.

Question: Please describe what a patient would consider a miracle that you helped them with.

Dr. Lewis:　　　My very first exposure was back in 1995. A patient came in a wheelchair, and she couldn't hold her head up. It was bobbing back and forth, and she couldn't get the insurance companies to give her a wheelchair that had head support. They told her that she could have brain surgery, but they wouldn't pay for anything to stabilize her head. I'd prayed to God to send me a miracle case. Everybody has a miracle story, and I wanted my own. When she came in, she asked me for help and I told her, "I have no idea what we're going to do, or if it's going to work, but we're going to do it, and we'll jump in head first if you'll just do everything I ask you to."

We took a look at her neck x-rays, and we did food sensitivity testing, IDG. We pulled her off nearly 20 plus food sensitivities. We did her blood chemistry and looked at where her nutritional deficiencies were and after all that, we adjusted her neck. Within two months, she was out of the wheelchair and perfectly healthy.

Her insurance wouldn't pay for chiropractic; they wouldn't pay for the nutrition, but would give her brain surgery if she wanted.

Question: Can you share a lesson you learned early on that still impacts how you run your practice today?

Dr. Lewis: Yes. I practiced under a doctor for three years before I went out on my own in 1988. I took a practice-building course. There I was, a young lady scared stiff, first time on her own. I was told to put the patients face down, and take all the waiting chairs out. When the patient was face down, I was to walk in the room, adjust them, and leave. I tried it all of one day. The next day I said, put all the chairs back, patients go face up. I'm here to see people and get people healthy, not to treat the back and disappear. I want to have a relationship with the patient. I want them well. I learned head-on that if you're going to survive in this business, you better be passionate, and you better love your patients.

Question: There are plenty of health benefits from using a chiropractor. Can you talk about a few of those benefits?

Dr. Lewis: The one thing I tell my patients and my Medicare patients is that when Medicare tried to get rid of chiropractic in the early 90s, they did a study. They paid Rand

Corporation to find out how much money they we were costing them, and what they found is that Medicare patients who got one adjustment a month for maintenance care had a 40% lower health care cost-including their chiropractic-than those who didn't.

Question: What are some myths and misconceptions that people have about chiropractic?

Dr. Lewis: The big one is that chiropractic causes strokes. If you look through Texas history, there has not been a single case dealing with a chiropractic causing a stroke. If you look at the numbers, back in 1988, the risk for a stroke was 1 in 1.75 million adjustments. I now know from Dr. Scott Haldeman, who's an MD, PhD, and chiropractic out of Canada, that the risk for stroke was 1 in 8.06 million in 2014. The risk for dying from an aspirin is 1 in 30,000.

Question: Any other myths or misconceptions that come to mind?

Dr. Lewis: That you have to keep going. It's kind of like the dentist. Once your teeth are clean and you feel that sheen, you know they're good, so why would you never go back again? You do maintenance care every six to nine months. I do the same thing with chiropractic. Once you know how great your body feels when it's totally lined up, in tune, and working properly, why would you let that feeling go, you're investing in yourself?

Question: What are some of the common fears people have about chiropractic?

Dr. Lewis: People think it's going to hurt. I'll tell you right up front at the first adjustment that it may or may not hurt. You have a chance of it hurting if you've been out of alignment for years or if you tighten up when we try to go to adjust you, but usually it's very simple. The example I use for patients is when you go to the gym. If you and I went out to the gym right now and we worked out, the next morning when we got up, if we were feeling like a million bucks, that would mean we're in good shape. If we woke up that next morning and were sore all over, guess what? Does that mean exercise was bad for you, or we're out of shape?

The same thing applies to chiropractic. If we are sore in the morning, does that mean the chiropractic was bad for you, or that you were out of alignment for a long time? Be aware that it takes time to make a change. Just like braces take time to straighten your teeth, it takes a little bit of time.

Question: I'm sure you've had patients who were scared; can you describe a situation or two where you helped them overcome that fear?

Dr. Lewis: I start simply by checking their wrists, elbows, and shoulders and then make an adjustment if it's needed. They see how easily that is performed. It's pretty much painless. I do that with all my patients. I start with something simple. They teach you to go right to the area that's causing a problem. You know that area is going to be sure, it's going to be a problem, and so you go to other areas. I prefer to go to other areas that are tied to the problem area, like the elbow or shoulders if it's a neck problem. Always make sure that they're comfortable with what you're doing.

Question: What's the one thing we haven't covered that you want to share with someone who is considering chiropractic?

Dr. Lewis: It's probably going to be the best investment you've ever made in your life. Don't just plan on going once. I've had patients that come in one time and they think everything's going to change. It's like putting braces on your teeth for one week and saying, "Oh, my teeth are better now." Make a long-term investment in yourself and your health. We can help a person live healthier longer.

Question: How can someone find out more about you?

Dr. Lewis: Go to my website or just call the office. My staffs are firm believers in chiropractic. I hired a Godly Christian staff. Just punch in Dr. Doreen Lewis, San Antonio, Texas, and it should come up. The website is: http://chiropractic-sanantonio.com/

CHAPTER TEN

Dr. Morgan Oaks

An Evolution in Chiropractic

DR. MORGAN OAKS

Dr. Morgan Oaks is a practicing chiropractor in Seattle, WA. He is also an international teacher and speaker whose passion is empowering people in every facet of their life. Over the course of his career, he discovered that optimum physical health is just one component to a balanced and vibrant life. His goal is to help people see the bigger picture, to figure out what they want, and give them the tools to live the amazing life they have envisioned.

Conversation with Dr. Oaks:

Question: Tell me about your practice and the patients you serve.

Dr. Oaks: My practice is highly varied. The people I see are of all ages and all walks of life. The youngest patient I've seen was three days old, and the most senior was a 93-year-old woman. The 93-year-old woman used to come in with her 67-year-old daughter so they both could receive care. The 67-year old woman was experiencing no pain. She simply wanted to become healthier so that she could hike all the trails in the Hawaiian Islands.

Initially, some people only want to get out of pain and regain normal function. After discovering what life can actually feel like, many of my patients continue with care as a way to maximize their health, and it is these patients who utilize chiropractic for preventative healthcare.

Question: Do you specialize in anything in particular?

Dr. Oaks: I believe my specialty is seeing the bigger picture of health - from a holistic point of view - and to help my patients in ways they specifically need to be helped. The lives people lead are too advanced to be able to apply a one-size-fits-all approach. I'm always diversifying the ways in which I support my patients.

When I was going through chiropractic school, I trained in the physiotherapy department, which integrated strengthening and stretching muscles with what I was doing with chiropractic. My first four years in practice were focused on changing my patient's posture in addition to providing muscle work and traditional chiropractic adjustments. I have also focused on treating athletes and working with injuries and dysfunction of the arms and legs. I add more to what I do every year.

At this point, I'm really focused on empowering people to do everything they can to take care of themselves. If dentists didn't teach us about the toothbrush and floss, they would be doing us all a huge disservice. I think in chiropractic and all healthcares, it's the same.

The more I can empower my patients to do on their own, the healthier and happier they are going to be both short and long term. I educate them on stretching and strengthening specific muscle groups, general exercise, ergonomics, postural change, diet, supplementation, and stress reduction. The more my patients can do for themselves, the better the results they will get from my care.

Question: How have you made a difference in the lives of people who come see you?

Dr. Oaks: Changes in the lives of my patients are as varied as the people themselves. In general, there are two types of people that tend come into a chiropractic office: people that are trying to escape pain, and those that are trying to improve their overall health and maximize their experience of life.

The first type of patient might have low back pain, neck pain, or headaches that are negatively impacting their life. What these people want is to get out of pain so that their life can return to normal. That's certainly why a large percentage of people initially turn to chiropractic, and chiropractic does a great job of helping these patients get out of pain.

More specifically, I've seen the following things occur with this first type of patient: a patient would come in for a migraine and the headache would be gone before she left. Another patient would come in for vertigo and it would improve within minutes of the treatment. I've also helped three separate people who had between three and six foot surgeries yet were still experiencing pain. All three people were able to experience vast improvement in symptoms and a return to specific activities and types of footwear. These results are great to be a part of, but the best part of practicing chiropractic is proactively supporting healthy lifestyles.

The majority of patients I see are on the other end of the spectrum; they're looking to maximize their health and experience of life. Many patients who come into the office hoping to get out of pain end up continuing care for this reason as well. This group isn't typically experiencing any pain, but through chiropractic care and lifestyle changes they may experience increased energy, a stronger immune system, or improved strength and flexibility. They may sleep better or find that they no longer suffer from reoccurring sickness or injuries. They also find resolution with issues they have experienced most of their lives. These patients experience real and lasting positive changes in their lives that they never expected from their chiropractic care.

Question: What made you decide to become a chiropractor?

Dr. Oaks: That's an interesting story. I never planned on being anything more than a chiropractic patient. I had a football injury in eighth grade where I got hit on top of the head during an onside kick. By the time I got home, I wasn't able to turn my head left or right. The next morning, my mom took me in to see her chiropractor to get an adjustment. After the visit, I was immediately pain free with a full range of motion. The only downside to the experience was that 30 minutes later I was back in school.

From that point forward, I received chiropractic care for all of my sports injuries. I thought getting an adjustment at the end of a season when I had no pain was preventative care. I continued to see a chiropractor all through high school and during the four years I played rugby at the University of Wyoming.

While I was working toward my degree in mechanical engineering, I realized that I didn't want to be stuck in a cubicle for the rest of my life. During Christmas break of my junior year, I looked into leaving engineering school to become a chiropractor. I eventually decided I would earn my engineering degree, finish what I had started, and find a job that made me happy.

A few years later, I was working in Denver, Colorado at an engineering firm. I was already referring friends and family members to chiropractic and they were getting good results. I continued getting adjusted while I played for Boulder's Rugby Football Club. I finally decided that to become a chiropractor and start providing the care that had been so beneficial to me and many of my friends and loved ones.

Question: Do you have any stories of patients you've treated whose results seemed miraculous?

Dr. Oaks: As part of our education, we're given the opportunity to travel abroad and give free chiropractic care around the world. For my clinic abroad, I went to Fiji. At these clinics, you end up seeing people that, in the United States, probably would have received care weeks, months, or even years earlier. In Fiji at that time, health care availability was limited and we ended up seeing a number of people with some very interesting issues.

One of the patients I saw in Fiji was a two-year-old boy that had never slept more than four hours at a time. He also had never walked, and was, in general, a disgruntled little boy; not very healthy, and not very happy.

His family brought him to the clinic to get treatment. As I worked on him, I determined that both his neck and his pelvis were not moving properly. The boy cried and fussed before the treatment started, and continued until his neck adjustment. Immediately after his adjustment, he calmed down completely and became very quiet and content. I also adjusted the rest of his spine and hips. He was asleep in his mother's arms before they left the clinic.

The next day, his mom brought him back to the clinic, and his whole family lined up outside and peered in through the windows. His mother told us that after the adjustment the day before, her son slept for four hours during the afternoon, slept all night, and had walked for the first time. I adjusted him again, and he was able to walk for us there in the clinic.

I'm certainly not saying that he never would have walked without chiropractic, but if you're not able to get sensory input from your body up to your brain, it makes it hard to learn those first steps. It was a huge blessing to be able to work with him and to see such immediate results.

I also hear many stories in my own clinic of people that have given up hope. There was a man that came to my office a couple years ago for low back pain. In the paperwork, he was asked about other issues and he mentioned that he had foot pain for quite some time. I asked about it further, and he said, "I've had foot pain since 1975." In my mind, I smiled and thought, "Wow, your foot pain's as old as I am!" I finished our health history and exam and got him adjusted. As he left the office that day, he said, "My foot hasn't felt this good in over 30 years!" I'm always amazed by the results that chiropractic can facilitate, and it's especially rewarding for those people who have given up hope.

Question: What is a lesson you learned early on that still impacts how you run your practice today?

Dr. Oaks: One of the biggest things that became evident when I got into chiropractic school was that a lot of chiropractors and students had really strongly-held beliefs about which chiropractic technique is best. There are so many effective techniques in chiropractic; they're typically named after the innovative doctors that had invented and developed them. I have devoted a lot of time to learning as many techniques as I can because they all get results, but not always in the same way, or with the same patients.

I was also interested in integrating healing modalities that might not fall under traditional chiropractic. Like I said before, I also worked in the physiotherapy department at school. It made sense to me that if you address the bones and joints directly with chiropractic, you should also address the muscles needed to help strengthen and stretch them.

I'm a big believer in looking at all the possibilities available to help a person, and to integrate and implement those possibilities in a way that makes the most sense for the patient. I address the bones, joints, and nervous system with chiropractic adjustments. I like to address the muscles with physiotherapy. I also give my patients things they can do at home, including stress reduction techniques and dietary changes.

Dietary changes and supplementation can make a huge change in the inflammation a person has in their body. Inflammation has a lot to do with pain. People initially come in as a way to diminish that pain, so if you can help them reduce the inflammation, a lot of the pain issues rapidly decrease, and we can then focus on the underlying dysfunction.

137

My goal is to look at the entire patient and their life, determine what the root cause of their issues is, and suggest the best ways to help them experience the life they want. Sometimes that is the care I provide, sometimes it is something they can do for themselves, and sometimes it is a referral to another provider. Their health and healing is always my main objective.

Question: What are some benefits to using a chiropractor that people may not be aware of?

Dr. Oaks: Before I entered chiropractic school, I had experienced five years of chronic heartburn. If I drank water or ate a banana, I got heartburn. If I had orange juice or spicy food, the heartburn was horrible. I was living on antacids. After getting regular adjustments for just a few weeks at school, my heartburn disappeared completely and I still have no symptoms over 15 years later.

It's important to understand that the brain and nervous system control everything that's happening in the body. If the information from the brain does not make it to the body, there will be a negative impact on that person's health. Chiropractic helps maintain clear communication between the brain, nervous system, and the rest of the body. For this reason, many people see positive results with chiropractic care well outside of back pain or headaches. It affects the whole body.

Many people do not realize that chiropractic can help for common ailments. I help patients with headaches, TMJ, neck pain, and back pain. I also adjust extremities, so I see people with carpal tunnel, tennis elbow, shoulder issues, knee pain, and plantar fasciitis. These can all be successfully treated with chiropractic care.

The most interesting results are when people have symptoms or issues outside of the spine or extremities. Patients report chiropractic having a positive effect on their asthma, vertigo, sleep, energy, bowel movements, digestion, concentration, and allergies.

I also work on pregnant mothers and children, although it's not a primary focus in my office. There are chiropractic offices where the entire office is focused on helping mothers who have struggled with fertility, helping breach babies turn, and ensuring that children develop properly. Colicky babies also see great results with chiropractic. There are so many different ways that chiropractic can positively impact a person.

Question: What are some myths and misconceptions people generally have about chiropractic?

Dr. Oaks: I think a lot of the myths out there are due to a lack of understanding or a bad experience. For most of us, if we have a negative experience with a dentist or a primary care physician, we find another doctor that fits our needs. It seems like for some people, if they have a negative experience with a chiropractor, they tend to write off the entire profession. All chiropractors (and doctors in general) are not created equal when it comes to patient communication, bedside manner, business practices, and setting an expectation for outcomes from treatment. It's important that all patients find a chiropractor that feels right for them.

One of the other misconceptions is that you have to have your neck rotated or for there to be popping in the spine during the course of care. There are many ways to provide chiropractic treatment and the popping and twisting of the neck aren't a necessity. There are many gentle ways to adjust the spine so that the body can heal on its own, and in my office, I make sure each patient receives care that resonates with them.

Another myth is that if you start seeing a chiropractor, you'll have to see one for the rest of your life. I always find this one a little amusing. No one would ever expect to go to the gym once, eat healthy once, or brush their teeth once and expect the results to continue indefinitely. The same is true with chiropractic care. Although many people find relief after one adjustment, regular visits to a chiropractor can prove beneficial toward living a healthy lifestyle.

The truth is, you don't need to go to a chiropractor forever. Just like you don't need to work out, eat healthy, or brush your teeth forever either. But we all know that by doing these things we will experience a healthier and happier life in the future. Some people choose to utilize chiropractic like an aspirin. They get care long enough to get out of pain, and then they stop coming until they're in pain again. It's not the best way to use chiropractic, and the body tends to continue getting worse over time if used in this way.

Question: What are some common fears people have about chiropractic?

Dr. Oaks: One of the fears goes back to neck popping. Like I said, there are many ways to provide great treatment that don't involve popping. People also fear the potential side effects of chiropractic. There's really no treatment out there that doesn't have a risk of unwanted side effects, and the risk for chiropractic is extremely low, even when compared to the common aspirin. Chiropractors perform a very thorough intake, health history, and exam before any care is given. We are trained to discover if a patient should not receive care or if they should be referred to a different provider.

Another concern patients have is that the chiropractic adjustments will make the joints too loose. This isn't an issue because the only joints a chiropractor will adjust will be the tight or restricted ones. The joints that move properly will be left alone. Many times a chiropractor will discover that there are joints that are already too loose, and exercises can be given to stabilize these areas.

Question: What's the one thing we haven't covered that you would like to share with someone who's considering chiropractic?

Dr. Oaks: I think chiropractic is a great healing modality to help people improve their lives, and often in a way that they didn't even expect. A lot of the people that I meet in my office have given up hope. Their diagnosis turned into a kind of life sentence, and they've given up on expecting anything different for their future.

Chiropractic care can create positive changes in a person's health and I believe chiropractors do a really great job on educating patients about their health in general. Educated and empowered patients can then create their own improvements by making small changes in their nutrition, exercise, posture, ergonomics, and/or mindset.

I always suggest family, friends, and patients use me as a health resource as well. If I'm not the provider who can help that person get well, many times I do know a provider who can and refer them directly. Chiropractors are also a great resource when a person has given up hope. If nothing else has worked, chiropractic may offer a solution to help them get their health and life back.

Question: How can someone find out more about you?

Dr. Oaks: The best place to find information about me and my office is through my website DrMorganOaks.com. The phone number is 425-444-4815, and the best email address is contact@drmorganoaks.com.

CHAPTER ELEVEN

Dr. Chris Michlin

Back to Health Family Chiropractic

DR. CHRIS MICHLIN

Dr. Chris Michlin is a licensed doctor of chiropractic serving the Dallas/Fort Worth, Texas community.

Dr. Michlin began healing people as a certified massage therapist in 1991. His clients experienced great relief, yet he realized that without correcting the underlying issue, the relief would not last long. Dr. Michlin knew that he needed to further his studies in order to help people get to the root of their pain and health conditions.

Dr. Michlin graduated in 2001 from Palmer College of Chiropractic in Davenport, Iowa. He uses an entire system of chiropractic care called the Palmer Package, which includes Gonstead, Thompson Drop, Derefield Leg Check, and Webster's Technique. He also uses the Sacral Occipital Technique (SOT), Cox Flexion-Distraction, and Activator Method.

Dr. Michlin is the only board certified Atlas Orthogonal chiropractor in North Texas. The results from an Atlas Orthogonal specific chiropractic adjustment are often immediate and dramatic. Dr. Roy Sweat, the founder of the Atlas Orthogonal procedure, is considered by many to be one of the foremost authorities in the world on the cervical spine.

Dr. Michlin was taught by Dr. Sweat, and he worked directly with him for his externship.

Dr. Michlin uses a "whole person approach". This approach to wellness means looking for underlying causes of any disturbance or disruption (which may or may not be causing symptoms at the time) and making whatever interventions and lifestyle adjustments necessary to optimize the conditions for normal function. Using this unique approach, Dr. Michlin is able to help the patient accelerate and/or maintain their journey to good health.

Conversation with Dr. Michlin:

Question: Please tell me a little about your practice and the patients you serve.

Dr. Michlin: Back to Health Family Chiropractic, LLC is a family owned and operated clinic. We meet our patients' individual needs and provide a WOW experience for each patient. Nancy, my wife and business partner, and I provide innovative wellness treatments that direct each patient towards his/her best possible health. When Nancy and I opened our practice, we had a concept that served as a foundation for all of our decisions, which is to do the right things for the right reasons.

As the only board certified Atlas Orthogonal doctor of chiropractic in North Texas, I provide a unique adjustment that is extremely gentle and specific to the top bone in the spine, the atlas. This is coupled with a wide range of full spine adjusting techniques. The atlas is extremely important, because it is the juncture where the brain meets the body. Even the slightest misalignment can create neurological miscommunication and dysfunction to any cell in the body. I also utilize specific full spine chiropractic techniques, provide soft tissue work, and targeted nutritional protocols to compliment the atlas orthogonal care.

Many of our patients experience chronic pain and have not gotten any relief from other healthcare providers. Those patients have experienced incredible results in our clinic. We treat auto injury patients as well as people who are suffering from chronic back and neck pain, headaches, migraines, neurological dysfunctions, and much more. I've adjusted patients from an hour old to over 100 years old. Our patients travel from all over the world to receive the atlas and full spine care that I provide.

Nancy has a Master's of Education degree in Instructional Systems Design and Technology. She's not only the CEO of our chiropractic and wellness clinic, she is also a wellness consultant, certified health coach, and motivational speaker on the principles of living a healthy lifestyle. Nancy implemented our sister company Back to Health for Life! Which focuses on four pillars of health and wellness: nutrition, exercise, stress reduction, and gratitude focus? Nancy's mission is to educate, inspire, and empower others to make healthy life choices to prevent disease or to learn how to flourish in spite of it.

Often the people that we serve have gone through the gamut of healthcare options before finding our clinic. A well-kept secret in healthcare is that by removing neurological interference at the source, we can enable the body to heal on its own without the need for dangerous medications and/or unnecessary surgeries. Many times, people come to us as a last resort after trying multiple doctors with no success. Part of the challenge is to overcome the side effects of previous treatments. Every person's body may respond differently and the effects on the body can vary, thus we help people who are experiencing a wide variety of health challenges.

Question: What are some powerful outcomes that you have helped patients achieve?

Dr. Michlin: We see miracles every day. For example, we had a patient who had an eight-week migraine that completely resolved after her first adjustment. We have seen people who are diagnosed with multiple sclerosis achieve complete resolution of their symptoms.

We helped a young lady who was diagnosed with dysautonomia. She was unable to attend classes at high school or even leave the house due to neurological miscommunication in her body. Her symptoms ranged from severe nausea, vomiting, diarrhea, and constipation to headaches, generalized pain, vaginal pain, and irregular, painful periods. Now, she attends college classes, goes to parties, and enjoys a much more normal life.

There was a six-year-old boy who could only walk on his tiptoes. He'd throw himself on the ground in fits. It took another doctor, his grandmother, and me two hours to get three pictures of his atlas. Although he understood normal communication, he could not speak with clear sentences or express his thoughts in a normal fashion. Immediately after his first adjustment, he had a whole body release and wet himself on the table. He then proceeded to stand up, flat-footed for the first time in his life. While walking back to help set himself up for the post cervical x-rays, he clearly told the office manager that he felt better.

Another outcome that stands out is a woman who spent 20 years seeing hundreds of doctors. These included a variety of specialists as well as taking medications and seeing a large variety of massage therapists, holistic doctors, and several chiropractors in search for answers to her fibromyalgia symptoms. She is also now living a normal, energetic, and pain free life.

While those are a few of the more extreme situations that we see on a regular basis, it is not even close to a comprehensive list. We're also very proficient in helping people resolve normal things that people think of with chiropractic care such as headaches, neck pain, back pain, scoliosis, and sciatica.

Question: What is a big problem that you specialize in solving?

Dr. Michlin: The main problem that we resolve is neurological dysfunction. By specializing and working in the region of the brain stem, we can solve a myriad of problems. We are able to help those suffering with migraines, trigeminal neuralgia (neurological face pain), fibromyalgia, Chiari syndrome, TMJ dysfunction, multiple sclerosis, and a variety of neuropathies.

To further discuss a direct example of the special problems that we help resolve, we can look at Chiari syndrome. Chiari malformation is when the base of the brain stem protrudes through the base of the skull. Chiari malformation can be congenital, meaning you're born with it, or it can be induced by a whiplash injury as can occur with a fall, sports injury, or in a motor vehicle collision. Due to the corking effect on the brain stem and the spinal canal, there's direct pressure on the brain stem as well as a physiological block in the cerebral spinal fluid circulation, normal blood flow, and lymphatic drainage from the brain.

Symptoms of the Chiari malformation include, but are not limited to, dizziness, vomiting, headaches, body aches, chronic fatigue, challenges with breathing, heart rate, difficulty swallowing, and generalized neurological dysfunction such as tingling, numbness, etc. Often Chiari malformation is not properly diagnosed and the symptoms are treated incorrectly. Let me briefly explain. The conventional diagnostic tool for a Chiari malformation is a recumbent, as in lying down on your back, MRI. Since gravity is always in effect, the brain moves slightly towards the back of the head and may open up the neural canal in that position.

A better, yet much less widely utilized tool is an upright MRI in which the patient is sitting and the gravitational force seats the brain back into the base of the skull. An additional consideration is that people who read MRIs are trained to disregard a Chiari malformation that protrudes less than 5 mm below the base of the skull. Food for thought: will air stay out of a bottle that is only slightly stopped by a cork any better than when the cork is pushed fully back into the bottle? Same question with cerebral spinal fluid in the brain. Pre and post upright MRI studies have been performed utilizing the upright Fonar MRI to show the brain can move back towards a normal position following an atlas orthogonal chiropractic adjustment.

These studies were conducted related to people diagnosed with multiple sclerosis and showed remarkable changes in the improvement of CSF flow, cerebral spinal fluid flow, healing of the brain, and reduction of related symptoms. The research is available at the official Atlas Orthogonal website, www.globalao.com or on Fonar's website, www.fonar.com.

Question: Describe the difference this outcome can make in a patient's life.

Dr. Michlin: People get their lives back. Many of the people who come to us have been in chronic pain for years. They've gone to many other doctors, spent a great deal of money, and were no better off. When their pain is eliminated, as a result of the care we provide in our clinic, they literally get their lives back.

Question: What made you decide to become a doctor of chiropractic?

Dr. Michlin: I was lucky enough to realize that I had the gift of healing hands early on and fortunate to have help in becoming a professional massage therapist 10 years prior to becoming a doctor of chiropractic. What I learned was that my clients felt better when they got off my massage table, yet their relief was not long lasting. They always had the same general issues. Tired of not getting more permanent results, I decided to learn more about the body and ways that I could get to the heart of the problem. Knowing that I did not want to cut people open or propagate the over medication of America, I searched for another avenue. Chiropractic was the natural direction for me.

Question: Can you share a lesson you learned early on that still impacts how you run your practice today?

Dr. Michlin: There are two major lessons that I learned early on which have helped shape our practice. The first one is that chiropractic is specific. Do not manipulate the spine. Give an extremely specific adjustment to the segment of the spine where the interference and nerve flow exists. By removing specific neurological interference, the brain and body can achieve clear communication. It is the clear communication between the brain and body that allows healing of the tissues to occur. The body heals from above, down, and inside out.

Number two is to not let insurance dictate care. By removing ourselves from the insurance system, we place the accountability of care where it belongs, between the doctor and the patient. People do not magically achieve health at whichever random visit insurance companies have decided they will cover. Each person is different, and each of our care plans are different too. As a side note, we do provide paperwork that allows for reimbursement from insurance companies. We believe each person should be able to collect the coverage for which they are paying; we just don't believe that an insurance company should dictate care.

Question: There are plenty of health benefits of using a chiropractor, can you talk about that?

Dr. Michlin: This is an amazing topic. Obviously, we can help with the general musculoskeletal aches and pains. The purpose of chiropractic treatment is not only to relieve pain, but also to improve quality of life by alleviating systematic problems within the body. The interesting part is brain and body communication. Since the brain ultimately controls every cell in the body, we owe all of our health to keeping the nervous system healthy. I'm not saying that there's never a time for medication and surgeries. When the body is overwhelmed or injured, we must use the appropriate treatment tools. With that said, a healthy body is designed to fight off foreign invaders and to heal wounds.

Well documented examples of how chiropractic care works to remove systemic interference and allows healing within us include the resolution of ear infections in children, lowering blood pressure by an average of 10 degrees Mercury, and a heightened immune response to infection causing fever. Amongst cancer survivors who seek chiropractic therapy, 84% do so to alleviate pain, improve mood, and sleeping habits as well as to relieve stress. The list of chiropractic side effects is extensive and of course varies with each person. Some of the more common effects of chiropractic care are better sleep, more energy, improved digestion, mental clarity, elevated sports performance, alleviated allergies, and asthma, increasing overall wellbeing, increased sex drive, balanced hormones, and reproductive system, improved healing, and stimulation of the immune system.

One of the best testimonies to a better health through chiropractic care comes from one of my younger patients.

When he feels a cold or a fever coming on, he tells his mother that he needs to go and see "the bone doctor". Mom happens to be a pediatric nurse who brings her children to our office to help boost their immune system. The boy and his brother do not get the traditional medicines and are very healthy. They have never had ear infections and are living a healthy lifestyle free of disease.

Of course, this works for adults as well. Many of our patients have discussed the decreased sickness, increased sense of wellbeing, and more robust lives that they are living as a "side effect" of regular chiropractic care. In essence, chiropractic care is a highly significant part of any program that is designed to help a person get and stay healthy.

Question: Let's talk about the myths and misconceptions people have about chiropractic. What are some of the more common ones that you see?

Dr. Michlin: You know I've heard some say that a chiropractor is not a real doctor. This myth is perpetuated by the medical field and popular media. In fact, it is well documented and easy to verify that the educational requirements for the medical doctor degree are less than the requirements for a doctor of chiropractic degree. This disparity of educational requirements exists both with the undergraduate hours required to pursue each degree as well as in the actual doctoral course work.

A Parker College study recorded that, on an average, chiropractic colleges require 372 more classroom hours than medical schools to attain a doctoral degree. Chiropractic students also have more hours of training in anatomy, physiology, diagnosis, and orthopedics (the musculoskeletal system). Beyond the basic coursework, there are also rigorous national and state board examinations in order to be licensed as a doctor of chiropractic. Like many of my peers, I've also put in thousands of extra classroom hours in order to pursue specialized studies beyond the basics of continuing education that is required to maintain licensure.

Question: What are some of the common misinformation and controversial topics about chiropractic?

Dr. Michlin: Currently and for many years the Texas Medical Association, TMA, has been suing the Texas Board of Chiropractic Examiners, TBCE, in the attempt to take away our legal ability to diagnose a patient's neuromusculoskeletal health conditions. When one considers the basis of education that is every bit as ludicrous as the TBCE suing the TMA in an attempt to take away the MD's right to prescribe medication. We have different areas of expertise and are better equipped to give specific types of care. Plain and simple, this is an attempt of the medical community to control every American's right to choose the care that best suits them. Meanwhile, more and more Americans are expressing an interest in ways to stay healthy instead of treating sickness.

Common misinformation is that chiropractic care is dangerous. Simply stated, I can lead the conversation by a discussion on malpractice insurance rates between medical doctors and doctors of chiropractic. Let's look at what insurance rates are based strictly on statistics. Anyone with a teenager behind the wheel knows that the insurance rates for teens are much higher than the insurance rates for an adult. This fact is due to the higher probability that the teenager will be involved in a motor vehicle collision than an adult. The same is true for malpractice between different kinds of doctors.

Utilizing the Cunningham Group statistics found at http://www.cunninghamgroupins.com/historic-medical-malpractice-insurance-rates/texas/, we could see that the rates in different areas of the state as well as for different specialties are very different. In an effort to level the playing field, I pulled up the most recent statistics from 2013 to compare the rates in our area. In Tarrant County, internal medicine doctors paid $11,997 to $21,254. General surgery doctors paid $34,744 to $58,430. OB/GYNs have the highest rates and paid $42,570 to $62,974 for their malpractice insurance.

My 2016 malpractice policy rate is $2,078. That means that three years ago the lowest risk, lowest paying doctors paid nearly six times as much as me and the highest risk and highest paying doctors in the same year paid more than 30 times as much for their malpractice insurance. Chiropractic care is not only safe, it is excellent for you.

Question: What are some of the common fears people have about chiropractic?

Dr. Michlin: What I hear the most is that people are scared of the noise associated with chiropractic adjustments and of being hurt. These are reasonable, but unnecessary fears. For one thing, the atlas orthogonal precision adjusting instrument delivers a completely painless adjustment with absolutely none of the noise associated with the traditional cervical adjustment. With that said, even when a doctor of chiropractic gives a traditional, specific chiropractic adjustment, there should be no pain. Yes, there may be some noise as the joints are moved and proper alignment occurs. This is normal and need not be feared. For those who have an absolute fear of the noise associated with traditional hand adjustments, I, and many of my colleagues, do offer alternative methods that are devoid of the sound.

Question: One of the questions that I'm sure you've heard is does chiropractic work? Or will my back be worse? How do you respond to this?

Dr. Michlin: Chiropractic works. I see it over and over with our patients. Are there pains associated? Yes. When we first start moving the spine, it's possible that your body's going to react. Neuromuscular pain, like the feeling you get when you've had a good workout, is common because muscles are shifting to hold the bones in the new position that we're putting them in.

Is it risky? You know, they've been trying to say that for many years. There was a study that came out in 2015 that showed the risk for stroke was higher if you went to a medical doctor than if you went to a doctor of chiropractic. When you look at those statistics, the chances are very low unless you are predisposed for a stroke in the first place.

The reality is that we don't hurt people. Again, this goes back to the malpractice insurance. If we were hurting people, our rates would be much higher and we'd have a lot more challenges. I tell people that they don't need to be scared, and we're here to help.

Question: How have you been able to help your patients overcome their obstacles?

Dr. Michlin: At our office we offer to waive the fee for the initial consultation, which allows me to sit down and discuss the person's situations and concerns. We discuss similar situations we've seen and how our care may help them. I describe the procedures that we use and introduce them to the Atlas Orthogonal Precision Adjusting Instrument. I'll walk over, put a finger under the stylus, and push the button that activates the instrument. I then have them put their finger under the stylus and let them feel what an adjustment will be like. In the words of one my younger patients, "that tickles".

On our website, BackToHealthTexas.com has a plethora of information. People can educate themselves on what services we provide at our clinic. We have a wonderful eight minute video about the Atlas Orthogonal adjustment and the instrument. We believe that education is our best way to help others make informed healthcare decisions. We also have abundance of patient success stories, both written and in video. Hearing other people discuss their experiences and great results speaks volumes to someone seeking care. It helps set his or her mind at ease and alleviates concern.

Question: What's one thing we haven't covered that you would like to share with someone who's considering chiropractic?

Dr. Michlin: Many people come to us when they're in pain. While that is certainly a great reason to seek chiropractic care, another great reason is to maintain good health. We change our car's oil every 3,000 miles to maintain its engine, we need to consider body maintenance too. The immune system interacts directly with the nervous system, affecting overall health. Again, obstructions with the signaling pathways between the nervous and the immune system impact the ability to heal adequately. Without the use of surgery or medication, chiropractic care removes these barriers so that the body can properly repair itself at a genetic level and fully stimulate the immune system.

159

For those who believe that staying healthy is expensive, I've got to ask this question, have you priced cancer lately? Prevention is far less expensive than illness. Great health takes a little bit of commitment every day. When we wake up each morning we make a decision about how we face that day, what we eat, our physical activities, and our mood. We're an embodiment of those choices. A person who saves money has more money. A person who saves health has greater health. Barring unforeseen incidents, the savings we bear will directly reflect the daily actions that got us there.

In the case of our health, we must consider that the brain and body work together in order to maintain homeostasis. Since the brain regulates every cell in the body, it is imperative to maintain clear communication lines between them. This is the job of the chiropractor. Chiropractic care helps people stay healthy and avoid illness.

Question: How can someone find out more about you and get more information about the benefits of chiropractic?

Dr. Michlin: We are very easy to find. Our website is BackToHealthTexas.com. Our address is 6324 Camp Bowie Boulevard, Fort Worth, Texas 76116. Our phone number is 817-810-9111. Our email is michlin@backtohealthtexas.com

CHAPTER TWELVE

Dr. Andrew Waitkevich

DR. ANDREW WAITKEVICH

Dr. Waitkevich received his Bachelor of Science degree in sports medicine/exercise physiology from Merrimack College in North Andover, Massachusetts. From there, he attended New York Chiropractic College where he graduated with Phi Chi Omega honors. He was awarded the Health Center Award at graduation and selected to participate in a highly competitive internship program during his final year of graduate education.

Dr. Waitkevich focuses on the conservative management of acute and chronic spinal and muscular disorders. He has a particular interest in sports chiropractic and muscular therapy. Recently, he concluded a postgraduate course to earn sports specific credentialing as a Certified Chiropractic Sports Practitioner (CCSP). Dr. Waitkevich is certified in Graston Technique, which is used to treat a variety of soft tissue disorders.

He currently holds active licenses to practice in Pennsylvania and New Jersey as a board certified chiropractic physician. He also holds adjunctive procedures certification in Pennsylvania. He is an active member of the American Chiropractic Association and its affiliated sports council.

Conversation with Dr. Waitkevich:

Question: Please tell me about your practice and the patients you serve.

Dr. Waitkevich: I maintain a part-time practice in Philadelphia. I treat a variety of patients all the way from children to the elderly. I focus on neck and back pain, but my specialty is in sports chiropractic, so I see a lot of athletes, tri-athletes, football players, soccer players, etc. Mostly, they are looking for injury prevention, pain relief, performance enhancement, and so on.

Question: Is there a problem that you specialize in solving?

Dr. Waitkevich: Aside from the general neck and back pain, I tend to focus the majority of my practice on the soft tissue component of injuries. I feel that along with the spinal components, if we don't address the soft tissue, it is like treating the problem halfway. I feel like I have pretty good outcomes. A lot of people come to me primarily for soft tissue treatments because it seems to speed up the process and they get better, more long-term results.

Question: What are some outcomes that you help them achieve?

Dr. Waitkevich: We get them to feel better faster. They also recover a lot quicker from their day in and day out activities. A lot of my patients overcome some of their obstacles in the work place, but also in their extracurricular activities. They notice improvement in their quality of life, and in their activities by setting personal records. If they're a runner, they feel stronger. Through chiropractic care and soft tissue treatments, patients seem to get quicker results.

Question: What made you decide to become a chiropractor?

Dr. Waitkevich: A couple of reasons actually. I've always had a fascination with the spine. My sister was diagnosed with severe scoliosis, so she had to have a spinal fusion. Now she has two rods, eight hooks, and a screw in her back. After her surgery, my interest in the spine grew. I wanted to investigate an avenue where I could help people with back conditions without surgery

The second reason is because of an injury I had as a collegiate athlete. I was undergoing a lot of PT and rehab, which helped, but it wasn't enough. I was actually taking an alternative medicine course at my school that was taught by a chiropractor. As I learned, I realized that what he was saying could help me recover. So I shadowed him. He started to treat me, and he resolved my condition in a couple visits. I wasn't able to achieve those outcomes from four months of regular rehab. That was the nail on the head right there; that's what told me that I had to investigate this, I had to look into chiropractic work, and what motivated me to go into this profession.

Question: Can you share a lesson you learned early on that still impacts how you run your practice today?

Dr. Waitkevich: In the beginning, when you first start practice, you want to think you can help everybody, but the biggest lesson I learned was to know my boundaries, and my limits. If there's a condition that is out of my scope, I'm confident that I can get the patient to the proper physician. Sometimes chiropractors develop a bad reputation because a lot of people think, "Oh I go to the chiropractor and they say they can treat everything," I think that can lead to problems down the road because if we think we can treat everything, there's going to be that one case that walks into your office that you think you can help and you could actually hurt the patient more. I think that's the main thing, knowing my limits. Being able to recognize things that I can help, and being able to point the people in the right direction if I can't.

Question: How long did it take you to figure that out?

Dr. Waitkevich: Within the first year. When you're in school, and learning about all the conditions its one thing, but when they're physically working in your office, it's a little different. Education is designed to get you to learn about it, but being able to see these people face to face, I think you develop that pretty quickly.

Question: What are some health benefits from using a chiropractor?

Dr. Waitkevich: There are lots of benefits to chiropractic. It goes beyond pain relief, it's all about performance enhancement, feeling better, and leading a better quality of life. Nutrition is a big aspect, too. I tell everybody when they come in with pain, "We get you out of pain, but diet and exercise is going to be what keeps you out of pain." We like to use a whole body approach. We get people better, get rid of their symptoms, but also encourage better activities, social activities, to eat better, exercise more, and avoid things that can contribute to their conditions.

Question: As far as myths and misconceptions about chiropractic, what are they and why are they wrong?

Dr. Waitkevich: A lot of people, especially people that are doing it for the first time, the common question they all seem to ask is, "I was a little hesitant going to the chiropractor, some other people I know said that once you go you have to always go." I think educating the patient is really important. Like I tell everybody, too much of anything is usually not good for you. We have to develop a program where we get rid of pain, get you on the right track, and then get you to the point where you're able to function, and do things on your own. Then we only bring you back in if needed, or if you have a setback. I also tell people that a chiropractor, any physician is really, is there to do 50% of the job, and that's to point the patients to the right path to what else they need to do to get the maximum benefit.

Question: What is some common misinformation that you've heard about chiropractic?

Dr. Waitkevich: The risk of stroke. I don't think there's enough research in that category, but people have a lot of fear when it comes to the chiropractor, and neck manipulation. I think if we had more research, people would understand that the risk is really low. It's very safe. There's a greater risk of injuring the neck if you go to the salon, lay your head back in extension, and get your hair washed in the tub, than getting a neck manipulation. It all comes down to technique. You have to be confident in what you do, make sure that you're doing it right, and that you're within the guidelines. Your patients should see the confidence in you, and they trust you.

Question: What are some common fears that people have about chiropractic?

Dr. Waitkevich: I guess they're not sure if it's going to work for them, if they're going to have to go for the rest of their life, or if the manipulation is going to cause more problems.

Question: Do people think that the side effects are risky?

Dr. Waitkevich: Yes. That's where I think going back to educating the patient is important. When I get new people in my office, I tell them that it's possible to be sore after your first couple treatments. Giving them the heads up, rather than just coming in, and performing the manipulation. Then they go home, notice they're sore, but nobody told them that they might happen. Then they get a negative depiction in their head, and sometimes that scares them away. If they know that ahead of time, that takes away some of those misconceptions.

Question: How have you helped your patients overcome their obstacles?

Dr. Waitkevich: My practice is part-time, and it's word of mouth and referral-based. I get a lot of older patients that have climbed the ladder as far as steps dealing with back pain, that have taken it all the way to the level of surgery, and they still have pain. They use the chiropractor as a last resort. I treat them within the limits, and boundaries that we're able to, depending on what their condition is, and they get relief. Some of those patients, they look me straight in the eye and say, "If I only knew what chiropractors did I would have come here first because I could have probably avoided a lot of the stuff that I did over the past however many years".

Question: Isn't that something?

Dr. Waitkevich: I see that a lot over here. It tends to be more of the older generation. People in their 50s and 60s that had herniated discs, but back in the day there wasn't enough knowledge or education about what a chiropractor does. They wouldn't get recommended or referred to see them, so they would go to PT. The PT would help, but the pain was still there, so then they tried injections, and when they didn't work, they had surgery. Post-surgery, they still have symptoms, they still have back pain. I think that's starting to change in today's world. We're getting a lot more medical referrals, and people are starting to understand that chiropractic is good. People are benefiting from it and it's helping cut healthcare costs, because if we can get people out of pain conservatively, it's going to help in the long run.

Question: What's the one thing we haven't covered that you want to share with someone who is considering chiropractic?

Dr. Waitkevich: Research. If somebody that's considering chiropractic is unsure, research and learn about both the benefits and risks. Knowing that it's safe, effective, and it's going to benefit them in the long-term can alleviate some of the fear.

Question: How can someone find out more information?

Dr. Waitkevich: I have a website: waitkevichchiropractic.com. There's a lot of useful information on there. I'm affiliated with some of the big chiropractic organizations: the American Chiropractic Association, the Pennsylvania Chiropractor Association, and the Sports Council.

My office phone is 215-969-2424. I'm normally available, and check my messages all the time. My email is waitkevichchiropractic@gmail.com.

Dr. Mitchell Pearce

DR. MITCHELL PEARCE

Dr. Mitchell Pearce is a graduate of Palmer College of Chiropractic –West class of 1989 and a 1990 graduate of the American College of Traditional Chinese Medicine. Dr. Pearce is board certified in nutrition by the American Board of Clinical Nutrition, which certifies medical, osteopathic, and chiropractic doctors. In 1983, Dr. Pearce was certified in sports chiropractic. Dr. Pearce is also a craniopath. Dr. Pearce has practiced over 30 years and taught in both chiropractic and acupuncture colleges. He currently teaches risk management courses to chiropractors and acupuncturists.

Conversation with Dr. Pearce:

Question: Please tell me about your practice and the patients that you see.

Dr. Pearce: My patients are those who have been unable to get well with other doctors, usually Western medicine doctors. They come to me for chiropractic, acupuncture, herbs, and nutrition. We find the cause of their illness, we treat the cause, and they get better. Many times, part of the cause is the various medications they've been taking. Prescription medications are often what bring them in.

Question: Are you known for a specialty?

Dr. Pearce: Well, I'm both a chiropractor and an acupuncturist. I'm board certified in nutrition. My services tend to be far more global. I also used to be a professor of both acupuncture and chiropractic.

Question: Do you specialize more in acupuncture or not necessarily?

Dr. Pearce: I'm a better chiropractor than an acupuncturist. When it comes to acupuncture, I primarily treat asthma and gastrointestinal problems, also some forms of arthritis, but my main focus is gastroenterology and pulmonary illnesses.

Question: What kind of success rate do you have with acupuncture?

Dr. Pearce: It's pretty good. Some people, if they've been on steroids for long enough, there's not too much I can do. Usually patients are able to get off steroids, able to breathe, and run up hill and play with all the other girls and boys. Sometimes the problems are allergic in origin, so I find the underlying allergy and then strengthen their immune system. In the Western model, there's this substance that causes you to be allergic, supposedly. In the Eastern model, there may be a triggering substance, but the problem is that your own system is weak, so it's overreacting to normal substances in the air or what you eat. I strengthen your system and then your body doesn't overact so you don't have allergic reactions. It's a very different model than the Western approach.

You could say the allopathic approach is to attack the vector, whereas the traditional Chinese and chiropractic approaches are to strengthen the host so much that the vector cannot attack the host. That's a fundamental difference between allopathic medicine, which is primarily based on trying to eliminate symptoms, to a traditional style of medicine, chiropractic or acupuncture, which tries to find the cause. If you have a pinched nerve in your back that's causing problems in your legs, arms, gallbladder, or spasms in your intestines, all the drugs in the world will never cure that. You have to cure the cause.

That's a fundamental difference. Admittedly, neither chiropractic, nor acupuncture, nor allopathic medicine can cure all illnesses alone. There are some things that Western medicine does pretty well, and for those patients, I send them to the appropriate doctors. In other cases, working together as a team is the only viable approach.

Question: What made you decide to become a chiropractor?

Dr. Pearce: When I was in college I had foot pain and a fallen arch. I went to an orthopedist and he told me that arches don't fall, that the foot pain must be in my head. I was hobbling around in foot pain for more than a year. Later, when I dropped out of college and I was living on the road--I was what people now call homeless--I was run over by a truck. I was sleeping on a lawn, the guy decided to park on the lawn, and so he parked on top of my knees. He drove over both knees and when he realized he was driving over me he panicked, shifted back into first gear, and drove back over me. I'm the only person I know who's been run over by the same truck twice.

I was taken to the local hospital. It was a rural area in Maine. There were 10 bed hospitals run by an orthopedic surgeon. I met him in the emergency room, and he told me I would never walk again if I did not have surgery immediately. I told him that he did not want to operate on me. After asking who the President of the United States was and becoming satisfied I was in my right mind, he asked, "Why don't I want to operate on you?" I said, "Because I've only got $75 to my name, $55 of it is in a bank account I opened two days ago, and I live in a tent in the woods. There's no way I'm going to be able to pay you for all this care." He said, "You're right, I don't want to operate on you." I made an agreement with him to buy two braces and rent a pair of crutches all for $70.00. He gave me some pain pills and I left the hospital on crutches.

I was driven back to where my tent was and fell asleep. I woke up, at least a day later and it was raining. I realized that if I stayed there, I would die from lack of food. Also, I could not stand up because my knees were locked straight in the braces. It took me two days to break camp, and put everything away, scooting around on my butt. I pulled the backpack up on a rope over a tree branch, and leaned the crutches in the crotch of the branch. Then I shimmied up the tree with just my arms and got the crutches underneath my arms. From there, I crutched to my hanging backpack, slipped the straps over my shoulders, and untied the rope. After stowing the rope around my waist, I crutched out to the street.

Two women in a station wagon picked me up. One of the women was a Native American medicine woman. She took me to her tepee. I know this sounds impossible, but it all happened. She took me to her tepee, and I stayed with her for two weeks. She filled me with herbs, and wrapped my legs with them. The herbs knocked me out, so most of the time I was asleep. After two weeks she said, "Okay, it's time for you to see if you can stand up." I stood up, still with the braces on, but now I could bend my knees a little. I could get myself up from lying down without having to shimmy up a tree. That was a major deal.

Then, she took me around on her house calls and saw that I was able to ambulate. She said, "Okay, you can go now. Here are the herbs you need to keep wrapping around your legs, use them up, and you should be fine. You'll eventually be able to do exercises for your knees and they'll recover." I've been able to do anything I want on my legs ever since.

That piqued my interest in herbal medicine. I decided to become a naturopath. The day I filled out my naturopathic application, I had a dream that my low neck cracked. At the same time, my girlfriend rolled over and hit me on that spot on my neck. I woke up unable to move and by unable to, I mean, literally unable to do anything. I was in tremendous pain. It was actually more pain than when I was run over by the truck. My girlfriend said, "Oh, don't worry about it. This used to happen to me all the time before I went to a chiropractor. Just go to a chiropractor and you'll be fine." Well, the problem was that I couldn't get out of bed. I tried to get chiropractors to make house calls and nobody would.

Three days later, I was carried into a chiropractic office by two people-literally carried in. He examined me, took an x-ray, adjusted my neck, and I was able to walk out. That was really impressive. When I was 16, five boys and I were in a collision with a police car. The policemen ended up in the hospital, both cars were totaled, and we all were sent home. The deal was that if we promised not to sue the police for running into us without lights or a siren, and they'd let us do anything we wanted until we were 21.

All of us agreed that we would leave the police alone and they would leave us alone. The result was that I didn't have any treatment for my whiplashed neck. Later when I was in San Francisco, after painting ceilings for several days, my neck finally had had enough and I ended up with a disc problem, which pressed on the nerves in my spinal cord and the nerve roots going up my arm. I was almost paralyzed. I could barely move. Anyway, the chiropractor treated me for quite a bit. At that time I was also really poor, but I owned a painting company that I had just started, and he agreed to let me paint his office for him in exchange for treatment.

Once I was able to get back up and running, I painted his office and became friends with him. He talked me into considering chiropractic instead of naturopathy. Also, during that period of time, every time I ate anything with fat in it I would throw up, have diarrhea, or get really ill. This had been going on for months, and I had seen lots and lots of doctors, Stanford doctors, UC San Francisco doctors, and the Haight Ashbury free clinic. I lived at Haight and Ashbury in San Francisco. This was in the 70s, at the tail end of the hippie era. Nobody could cure me. Nobody could figure out what was wrong. They even sent me to shrinks thinking that there must be something wrong with my head. The shrinks said, "There's nothing wrong with your head; there's something wrong with your guts."

Finally, I went to another chiropractor and he treated more of my neck. I still had some neck pain. The next chiropractor eliminated the remaining neck pain. Then, he said to me, "You turn yellow a lot, and every time you eat fat you get sick." I said, "How did you know?" He said, "Well, when I press here and here on your abdomen, these reflexes tell me your gallbladder doesn't work."

He said, "If you give me three to five visits, I'll make it so that your gallbladder will work and you'll be able to eat fat." At that time, I was 5'5" and under 105 pounds. I was really scrawny because if you can't eat fat, that's more than a third of your calories and you lose weight. I was pretty desperate. I thought I'd give him a try. He did some reflex massage and adjusted my upper spine, and upper back between my shoulder blades. On the third visit he said, "Okay, go out and have some fried eggs and bacon. I'll bet you'll be able to eat it and you won't have any symptoms." I went out and had breakfast. I had fried eggs and bacon and for the first time in more than a year, I could eat it.

That amazed me. He treated me some more and I was able to gain weight. Then, later he said me, "You know, your jaw is always tight and your head aches, I think I can fix that. I'm going to move the bones of your skull." I said, "Well, how much is that going to cost me?" He said, "Well, that's a specialty, I'll charge $35." In today's money, that would be $200 or so. On the third day he said, "Okay, your jaw is going to be pretty relaxed by the end of this treatment, but the other thing that happens with this is your vision may be a little different. I want you to walk home, relax, enjoy the day, and notice if your vision changes. Things may be a lot brighter."

I walked out of his office and things were way brighter, and more colorful. I don't know if you've ever seen one those Carlos Castaneda books where the covers are all pastel? When you go from pastel to full color, it totally blows your mind. That convinced me to become a chiropractor.

I called my parents to tell them that I was going to become a chiropractor. My mother burst into tears and sobbed on the phone. When my father was young, he was very rich, and brought up by a nanny. That nanny died of cancer. When she had back pain from her cancer, she went to a chiropractor and was made comfortable. The medical doctor for the family said that if she had not seen the chiropractor, they could have saved her.

Question: That had to have been hard.

Dr. Pearce: My father felt that chiropractors were murderers until the next part of the story. The doctors had no more ability to cure sarcoma then than chiropractors, but the chiropractors reduced her pain.

I went to Chiropractic College despite my parents' misgivings, worked my way through, and when I was an intern, there was this girl who was carried in by her mother. She was two years old, and unable to sit up. She had cerebral palsy. Her nose was constantly stuffed. She was asthmatic. She literally couldn't sit up let alone walk, or stand. She could barely talk because of her breathing difficulties. I treated her with chiropractic, and craniopathy, moving the bones of her skull and fixed her breathing issues, stopped all the ear infections, and stopped the mucus from pouring out of her. After about two months of treatment, I came into the office and she was standing in the middle of the room. She looked up at me, smiled, and said, "It's so easy."

179

When I graduated, that little girl came and sat with me; she just left her parents and sat on my lap with the graduating class. My father and mother had come to see me graduate, and my father thought, oh my God, he hasn't told us about having children! This child is two years old. He came to me and said, "Who's this little girl?" Then the parents of the little girl came up and told my father about how I had made it possible for their child to walk. That was the beginning of changing my dad's attitude towards the profession.

After all the festivities were over, he took me aside and told me that he had been diagnosed with cancer, and had less than six months to live. He had found that out and that's why he'd come to see my graduation. Over the ensuing weeks, I researched his cancer, and told him, "look at all the medical treatment for your cancer; all the studies have shown that medical treatment has no effect on making you live any longer, but it will make you feel a lot worse." He didn't believe that and insisted on going with the medical treatment, but he agreed to change his diet according to my suggestions. He changed his diet, and 15 years later he came into my office as a surprise. He flew across the country to say hi.

Fifteen years later, I looked at him and said, "Well, you look really good for a guy who was supposed to be dead 15 years ago." He burst into a smile and said, "Yeah, I'm still fooling them." He continued with the change in the diet that I had given him, and he out lived every single one of the doctors who told him he wouldn't live more than year. He was diagnosed at 62, and he died at 84 of pneumonia, not of his cancer.

Those are the kinds of things that made me into the kind of doctor that I am. Basically, the patients that I work best with are those who have gone elsewhere without success. What got me interested in gastroenterology problems was when I was in China. I didn't know that one of the peppers in the food was highly toxic if eaten. The locals all separated it from the food before eating. It damaged my intestines. I ended up getting sick, very weak, and lost 35 pounds. I was in Schezwan and the Schezwan pepper is in everything they eat, everything they cook. I didn't it realize it initially, because the doctors, not knowing I had not been told to put the pepper aside, insisted it couldn't be from the pepper.

It turned out that it was the pepper, and to make matters worse, I'd developed an allergy. I eliminated the pepper, took some herbs, and the gastroenterological problems went away. That made me interested in learning about food allergies, and food intolerances. I developed a specialty in that as well.

When I was in China, I became so ill and weak, that I developed asthma, bronchial asthma. I treated that with acupuncture and chiropractic. All of these different experiences motivated me to explore the specialties that I treat.

People with intractable migraines, headaches that have never been able to be fixed by anything else, in my entire career I've only had three patients with headaches that I have not cured. One was a girl whose father led with his left, and her skull was distorted from the amount of beatings she had suffered as she was growing up. One was a priest with migraines, and the other was a gentleman with cluster headaches, I wasn't able to cure. Everybody else I cured. The priest is the only one I didn't actually make better. The other two I made better, I just couldn't cure them.

The sicker a patient is, the more excited I am to take care of them. That's kind of where I'm at as a doctor.

Question: Is there a lesson you learned early on that still impacts how you run your practice today?

Dr. Pearce: Well, one is that some people cannot get to a doctor unless you do a house call. My entire professional life, I've done house calls. I'm the only doctor I know who still does. That's one thing I learned that impacts my practice. The other is not to turn anybody away for lack of ability to pay. The third is if you do the best you possibly can, and continue to learn, you'll get better and better at being a doctor.

Question: There are plenty of health benefits to using a chiropractor, can you talk about that?

Dr. Pearce: Well, I think the main thing is how underestimated and how undervalued chiropractic is. We've finally gotten over how it was when I first started, when you'd call a medical doctor and they'd hang up on you. Now, I call a medical doctor, they talk to me, and we can work together on getting the patient better. That's great as long as all I'm telling the doctor about is that this person's got a muscle spasms or a pinched nerve. There are a limited number of diagnoses that we've been accepted for. Really, the state and insurance companies, they won't pay us for all the other things that we do. Medicare won't cover it. Insurance companies won't cover it. State boards try to prosecute you if you're doing it.

Yet, that's where we do really. Also in general healthcare, just keeping a patient healthy. My younger boy has seen a medical doctor three times, when he was born, and two checkups, and one school physical, four times. That's it. He's eight years old. I've taken care of every illness for him. He's normally not sick for more than a day. All the other school kids are sick for three or four days, or a couple of weeks, with whatever are going around in the school. My older boy has had emergency care for croup, which is basically laryngitis, but in children it causes your larynx to swell so much that you have difficulty breathing. He ended up with emergency treatment for that, in the hospital, which literally saved his life.

The issue is that not everybody can cure everything, but we can do an awful lot more than what chiropractors are currently allowed to be paid for and sometimes even allowed to do. The attorney general here in California regularly harasses chiropractors who practice herbal medicine, even though it's in our scope. Acupuncturists practicing herbal medicine are a different story, because they leave us alone for that. Originally, chiropractic in California was actually naturopathy. It was chiropractic plus herbs plus nutrition plus any physical therapy. Chiropractic was a physical therapy license as well as a chiropractic license. That's still the case, but if you start putting herbs in there, the attorney general wants to prevent you from doing it.

That's kind of it in a nutshell as far as where things stand now, politically, in the profession.

Question: What are some of the myths and misconceptions people generally have about chiropractic?

Dr. Pearce: The most common misperception is that chiropractic is only good for headaches and neck, back, leg, and arm pain. It is very good for that, but the misconception is that's all we're good for. That's the single biggest misconception. People don't understand that all the smooth muscle in your body that controls your intestinal systems and the bronchi in your lungs are controlled by the nerves in your spine. If you've got a pinch in those nerves, those organs are not going to function right. Hence, a major cause of asthma, gastrointestinal issues, and irritable bowel syndrome, which then develops a leaky gut, which then develops allergies, which then develops Crohn's, and colitis. That's the progression for most of these illnesses. If you fix the spine, you stop that progression. You do acupuncture and herbs heal the gut mucosa, you fix the spine, you fix the cause, and you're done.

In China, this is just how they do it normally. This is the regular, every day, run of the mill treatment for Crohn's and colitis in China, standard of care. In the United States, the standard of care is to cut out your intestines piece by piece until you're unable to digest food, and you have to live on these formulas, which will never be as balanced as your food, you'll never be healthy, and you'll die young. That we are not recognized for what we are able to do in this country, which is standard medical practice in the largest population in the world, is very sad.

Question: What are some of the common fears people have about chiropractic?

Dr. Pearce: The single most common fear is that they're going to have a stroke from neck manipulation. The other is that we're going to break their bones. When they hear the popping sound, they think their bones are being broken, but they don't have any pain from the popping noise. People have this perception that chiropractors can twist your back, and break your neck. You really can't. I actually teach risk management for the State of California. I know these statistics by heart. The chances of having anything seriously go wrong during a chiropractic visit are less than 1 in 3.7

million. We're the safest profession in the world. It is physically impossible for a chiropractor to cause a stroke. There were claims, particularly by the Connecticut Society of Neurology; they made this whole advertising campaign about it. Attorneys have been trying to make a campaign about it because if you can claim that a chiropractor created a stroke, it's very lucrative for the attorney.

Physically, it's impossible. The artery that they're claiming has the stroke is the vertebral artery. What happens is that the arterial wall becomes weak because it's inflamed, and blood extravasates between the layers of the wall, pinching off the artery. They thought, well, if you're twisting the neck you're damaging the artery, you're pulling on it, but physically, we cannot twist the neck far enough to be able to stress the artery. The tests have been done in the last five years; the research has been done to prove that we simply cannot do it. It's not physically possible.

The cause of the stroke is inflammation of the artery, and I personally believe that inflammation of the artery is due to Trans fats. Trans fats are very inflammatory to the arterial wall. If you eliminate Trans fats, you don't get arteriosclerosis, and then you don't have these problems. You don't have any kinds of artery leaks, so to speak, that cause a particular kind of stroke. When the artery pinches itself off because it leaks inside the wall, and the wall presses back down onto the channel of the artery, it is what we call lumen. Basically, it shuts off the pipe, pinches off the pipe. That's how the stroke occurs. Research shows that normally, about 17% of people who have one of these situations happening in the artery that it has also been happening in smaller arteries that don't happen to be going to the brain. There's a new MRI technique that shows this. This is actually a manifestation of a general arterial wall inflammation, is what's truly happening.

Another fear is that we will cause a disc injury. Again, in order to injure a disc with twisting, you have to move with weight, and we're not doing that because the person's lying on their side for adjusting. If we adjust them sitting up there's weight, but they're lying on their side so there's no weight. You also have to twist. The research was done way back in the early 80s, and was published in the book by White and Punjabi, which used to be the standard textbook for medical surgeons in surgery of the spine.

Anyway, the bottom line is you cannot rotate the disc far enough to cause anything to rupture unless you cut off the back half of the vertebra from the front half. Only then can you rotate it far enough to do so. Well, we're adjusting whole vertebrae. We're not adjusting people who have had the back of their vertebrae removed, so it's physically impossible for us to rupture a disc. Nowadays, people who sue for a ruptured disc don't win. That's gone away as a threat to us in this profession.

I remember back in the 70s, 80s, and 90s, before this research became well known, it was a very common attempt against chiropractors. Most chiropractors, they'd see a patient with a bad disc, if the patient did not get immediately better, the patient would sue him claiming that he got worse. At one time there was a rate of 1 in 15 chiropractors at any one time dealing with that type of lawsuit. Now, they don't exist anymore because the research has finally become public knowledge in both the legal and medical communities. They know they can't win, and they know that if they sue a chiropractor, he might turn around and sue them for malicious prosecution, and that he'll win. That's gone away for the most part.

Question: What is one thing we haven't covered that you would like to share with someone considering chiropractic?

Dr. Pearce: There are many different ways that a doctor can manipulate the spine. There's virtually no chance that any chiropractor worth their salt, is going to manipulate the spine in a way that's going to hurt anybody. It's pretty much impossible to hurt anybody with it. I think the most important thing is that patients should not be afraid of chiropractors.

The next most important thing, and this may be more important, is that people regularly say that chiropractors performed a miracle. I couldn't walk, and now I can, and so forth, but to a chiropractor this is just another day in the office. This is something we do day in and day out. We see these kinds of "amazing results," like myself with the gallbladder problem, every day. All the stories that I told you are not unusual. The only thing that's unusual is that so many of them happened to me. Anybody who's had any of the experiences I've had or had children with the experiences that I've had, should go to a chiropractor. They'll get better. Their children might be able to walk. The child will end up having open sinuses, and be able to breathe. All of this stuff is just routine, every day, chiropractic results. It's nice to call them miracles because for people who are not chiropractors, they look like miracles. To us, it's ordinary science. It's as normal as walking from point A to point B.

Question: How can someone find out more about you?

Dr. Pearce: They can go to www.betterhealer.com.

CHAPTER FOURTEEN

Dr. Jason Kramer

DR. JASON KRAMER

Dr. Jason Kramer is the owner of Revolution Chiropractic. He grew up in the beautiful Pacific Northwest, just north of Seattle. He pursued his bachelor's degree in exercise science at Western Washington University while working at a local chiropractor's office.

Through his experience, he learned the science of chiropractic, but more importantly, the philosophy behind chiropractic.

Dr. Kramer graduated from Life University in Atlanta, Georgia. He has volunteered for multiple ministries and shelters, participated in National C.A.R.E. Day, and are an active member of the Plano Rotary Club.

Dr. Kramer is the biggest Seattle Seahawks fan in Texas. He looks forward to taking care of you and your family.

Licensed chiropractor in the State of Texas.

Conversation with Dr. Kramer

Question: Can you tell us about your practice and the patients you serve?

Dr. Kramer: We run a family chiropractic office here. We see everyone from little babies that are only a couple of days old to some of our oldest patients in their mid-90s. We're all about healthy families. We don't do any twisting, cracking, or popping in the office. It's very safe and gentle. In fact, parents that are apprehensive about bringing their children in for care quickly realize that it is not only safe and gentle, but necessary to have their children checked.

We focus on natural healthcare by treating the cause and not the symptom, which is why we're able to tell our patients that we expect them to get better. We use specific technology in our office that allows us to assess the nervous system, to locate areas of weakness, and correct them at the source, allowing the body to function and feel well.

We specialize in correcting nerve interference and obstruction, which is also called subluxation. The nervous system controls and coordinates every other part of the body, so we need that functioning the best that it can. Every patient that walks through our doors gets a full assessment. We treat each person individually.

Question: You mentioned treating infants that are only a few days old, what do you do with them?

Dr. Kramer: Ultimately, what we'll do is the same thing we'd do if they were older; we just do it in a different way. We assess them for any nerve interference; we check for different ranges of motion. A lot of it is talking with mom to see if the baby is breastfeeding, if that's going okay, if they've been colicky, if they've had any symptoms since birth. We ask these questions because we know that the entire birthing process can be traumatic for mom, but often we forget that the baby is going through that same experience. What end up happening are the symptoms and a problem the baby has gets written off as, "Oh, that's normal. That's a stage the baby's going through." While it may be common, it is not normal. We're able to assess those using ranges of motion and different objective measures that show us any areas of weakness or increased inflammation throughout the nervous system. After that, we're able to give small, gentle adjustments to allow the baby's body to work better.

Question: What difference have you made in the life of a patient that truly sticks out in your mind?

Dr. Kramer: That's a good question. We see such a wide range of issues in our office. We have people come in with severe dizziness, with blood pressure issues, with aches and pains, with asthma and respiratory conditions, and we help with a lot of those problem areas. It's difficult to pick one. Really what it all comes back to is that we're able to tell them that we expect them to leave better than when they came because we're going to treat the subluxated nervous system and make sure it's functioning at its best. If the nervous system is functioning well, the body's going to function well and feel well. All sorts of issues start to be resolved as long as that nervous system is fully intact and functioning.

Question: What made you decide to become a chiropractor?

Dr. Kramer: I've been asked that a few times recently, and I think it's a good thing to find out why your healthcare provider is doing what they're doing. I actually used to want to be a history teacher. The reason that I wanted to do that is because ... usually everyone can pinpoint a teacher or two throughout their lives that helped make a difference and make decisions in their life; I wanted to do that for other people. In addition, I'm a big history geek. I figured that that'd be a great way to impact people while enjoying what I do. I come from a big family, and that's just what we do.

I was treated by achiropractor when I was an undergrad for a car accident injury. He says to me one day, "Well, what are you going to do with your life?" Being a twenty, twenty-one-year-old kid, I figured that I had life figured out, which is never the case when you're that young. I told him that I wanted to be a history teacher. He said, "Well, if you're being serious, if you really want to change people's lives, if you want to give back, then you should be a chiropractor." I chuckled a little bit, which he didn't like. I told him, "I appreciate what you do. I know that you help people out of pain. I'm here because I was in a car accident, you're helping me with my neck, and I appreciate that. Helping people out of pain is a big deal, but I want to have a bigger impact."

194

He kind of gave me a weird look, as if he was about to scold me. He said, "You have no idea what you're talking about or what chiropractic is." He convinced me to come in and shadow him for a couple of days. By the time those days were over, man, I saw so much that I actually started working for him for free. I would go to school during the day, work for him three or four days a week in the afternoons, and then work nights stocking shelves just so I could be around him.

What I found was, yeah, people came in for aches and pains, but what was really cool was when I saw mamas bringing in their newborn babies. I saw moms getting adjusted throughout their pregnancy to ease and decrease the pain during delivery. I saw people coming off medications for allergies or blood pressure. I saw people come in with digestive problems and leave better. People coming in with all these different sorts of pains. I asked him, "What in the world is going on here?" He told me that the chiropractor has one job to do; correct any interference or obstruction throughout the nervous system (subluxation). The body's going to recover and heal like it was designed to do. Then we get the heck out of the way, and all this amazing stuff starts to happen. I was blown away. From that day forward, I knew I had to be a chiropractor.

Question: Can you share a lesson you learned early on that still impacts how you run your practice today?

Dr. Kramer: That's an interesting question because there were so many. One of the biggest things that I learned is that if we let a patient make their own care plan or schedule, they'll stop coming in as soon as the symptoms are gone; they'll think that they're better. The reason that's a problem is because now we're going based off of symptoms, and if you go solely based off of symptoms; you can't ever get to the root of the issue, whether it's aches, pains, sickness, disease, or general health concerns.

Running into those same patients down the road, they tell me, "Well, yeah, it helped for a little while, but you know what? Chiropractic didn't work for me." I realized it's not chiropractic that didn't work for them; it didn't work because they didn't stick to the care plan until that entire cause was corrected. So the biggest lesson I've learned being in practice is that you have to be the doctor. Take for instance a medical doctor. I mean, there's no medical doctor that would say, "Take whatever prescription drug you want and take it however often you want." There are very specific ways to do that, and it's done for a reason. That's the probably the biggest lesson that I've learned.

Question: Do you stress how important coming back to appointments is to your patients? Does that keep them coming back?

Dr. Kramer: We tell them that if they need to hear it. We're upfront about educating the patient and letting them know why we're delivering the adjustment. We let them know if they're coming in with neck pain, "I'm not treating your neck pain. I'm treating the cause of your neck pain. If we can get that corrected, your body's going to feel better, but it's only because it's functioning better. If we can make your body function better, I know it's going to feel better. It just takes time. It takes repetition. We expect you to get better, but the first thing that goes away is usually the symptom. We want to make sure that everything stays corrected." We explain the whole process so they have a pretty good understanding of what we do and how it should work.

Question: Obviously, there are plenty of health benefits to using a chiropractor. We'd like to raise awareness of the importance of seeing a chiropractor. Could you talk about some of these benefits?

Dr. Kramer: I think that's one of the biggest misconceptions about chiropractic and healthcare. Our entire healthcare system is based off of symptoms. You're told that if you feel good, then you're probably healthy. If you don't feel well, then go see a doctor. I think the biggest thing about chiropractic is that it can increase the entire function of your body. We like to talk about posture; we like to talk about the structure of your body because we know that proper structure will allow for proper function. There's a lot of correlation between deviations from proper alignment and proper posture and direct health conditions. So instead of treating a health condition, whether it is aches and pains or whatever else, we go back to posture and misalignments in the spine.

Question: What are some myths and misconceptions about chiropractic?

Dr. Kramer: I think the first one right off the bat is that people think that once you start going to chiropractor, you have to see him forever. We hear that a lot. In fact, even before people get started with care, they'll tell us something like, "Well, I don't really want to get started because I've heard that once you start, you always have to go." That is a complete misconception. My response to that is to always tell them that our ultimate goal is to get them corrected as fast as possible. If you want to talk about maintenance care afterwards, then that's great.

It's the same thing as going to a dentist to get a checkup. You wouldn't wait until you have a throbbing toothache and a huge cavity to see your dentist. You should be going for normal checkups. Same thing with eye care. You should see your eye doctor to check your vision and make sure everything is going well. That concept applies to the spine as well. You should check in with a chiropractor, in my opinion, every once in a while just to make sure everything's okay and to see if anything needs to be adjusted. You don't have to keep going forever, but I'm a huge advocate for checking in occasionally to make sure all is as it should be.

So it's not forever, but it is a, "Hey, every once in a while swing in and let's go ahead and get you checked."

I think another misconception is, "Why should I see a chiropractor anyway?" I get that a lot. I get, "Well, I hit the gym five or six days a week and I do yoga, so I don't really think that chiropractic could help." I think, "Well, that's great, you should be working out. That's important. Great and yoga's amazing." But that's completely different. You're comparing completely different things. Chiropractic is about addressing the spine and making sure that the nervous system is functioning at its best. Working out and doing yoga are going to be amazing for you and for your body, but they're aimed at completely different things. I think those are probably the two things that come up most often.

Question: Isn't another common misconception that people think you're going to a chiropractor to "get your back cracked"?

Dr. Kramer: You're right. We had that today. That's funny. Someone will, a lot of times, swing in for a "quick adjustment." "I just need a quick crack" is what they'll tell me. I'll tell them, "Well, crack's illegal here in our state. I'll do you one better. We're going to give you a specific adjustment, but we've got to get you assessed first." A lot of the time, they just haven't been educated properly. You can't swing in for a quick crack.

By the way, we don't do any twisting, cracking or popping here because our practice is much gentler, much more specific. If someone's coming in, usually when they want a quick crack or quick adjustment, they're coming in because of a symptom. So we explain to them immediately that, "Hey, you're coming in here because something is going on, causing pain. I don't want to adjust the area that's having pain. I'd like to find out why the area's having pain. See, if we treat that symptom, then it might feel good for a day or two, but we're not facing what's really wrong. Then you're going to leave and go, 'Man, chiropractic never works,' but that's only because you came in expecting to get your symptom addressed. What we want to do is find the cause of the pain."

Question: What are some of the common fears people have about chiropractic?

Dr. Kramer: Oh, probably the biggest one is that it's going to hurt. The other one is that chiropractic doesn't work. The hurt one, well, there might be some times where there's minor soreness after adjustments, but part of what we do without the twisting and cracking is allow your body to be in complete ease. As you're lying there before the adjustment, you don't get tensed up and worried that I am going to twist or pop something. That, a lot of the time, is going to put someone's mind at ease. Even if you did get manually adjusted, if it's done properly, there might be some simple soreness, just like if you hadn't worked out in a while and you hit the gym hard. Yeah, you can expect a little bit of soreness, but nothing pain-wise.

Question: How have you been able to help your patients overcome their fears of using a chiropractor?

Dr. Kramer: There are two main ways that come to mind. One is by education. If someone comes in, they're a little worried that it might hurt. They're a little worried it's not going to work. They're a little worried that ... a lot of times this is their last option. They've tried everything else. They want to know that it is possible to get help. It is unfortunate that the last resort is a natural form of health care like chiropractic. We're able to walk them through why the body responds in different ways. It's all about education. When they start to understand, they're much, much more comfortable with it. As opposed to going in blind and not sure of what's going to happen or why it's going to happen.

The other thing we get is people that think as soon as you start chiropractic care everything is going to go great from the beginning, that everything's going to get better every single day, and there's never going to be any setbacks. That's not realistic. We walk them through the process and let them know that occasionally there might be setbacks. It's like we're climbing a mountain. There are going to be peaks; there are going to be valleys. As long as we continue to climb, as long as we continue to ascend that mountain, we're going to reach the top. There may be minor setbacks that are okay. It's all part of the care. It's all part of the correction that's happening. As long as we keep moving forward, we're doing the right thing.

Question: So you find that when you educate your patients, it typically puts them at ease?

Dr. Kramer: Yes. People haven't been educated about what happens in the body, or why the body is reacting in certain ways, or how chiropractic can help. Educating them answers the and the *why*, allowing them to go in with full knowledge and understanding of what will happen. Getting rid of that uncertainty helps them relax.

Question: What's the one thing that we haven't covered that you would like to share with someone who's considering chiropractic?

Dr. Kramer: I think that overall health needs to be considered. We know full well that there's a time and a place for all different types of health care. We prefer to try natural care first. I think it, again, goes back to not only the education process, but also being objective with health care and with each individual. If you can eliminate the guessing when it comes to someone's body and target specific areas, with measurable results, then you can see why someone is going through different health issues, and why their body is acting the way it is. I really think what we should be getting away from is the idea of bad genes and bad luck leading to bad health. I really think that's just bad science and bad logic and leading to even worse health care throughout our nation. If we can educate people and be objective in our treatments, then we can measure and re-measure with expected outcomes and start to change communities.

Question: How can someone find out more about your practice?

Dr. Kramer: Go to our website at revolutionchiropractor.com. We also have a Revolution Chiropractic YouTube site and a Facebook page. All three have multiple sources of knowledge about chiropractic, how to locate us, and a little more about the practice itself. You can even learn more via our snap chat, username chirochat.

CHAPTER FIFTEEN

Dr. Amber Bloom

DR. AMBER BLOOM

Dr. Amber Bloom, a Chiropractor based in Texas and licensed in multiple other states, brings her experience inneuromusculoskeletal problems to a chiropractic practice of natural healthcare. Dr. Bloom provides a program of care designed to improve physical function and alleviate pain.

Dr. Bloom uses the latest innovative technique 'specific prone', a light, gentle, and comfortable technique with outstanding results. She also specializes in the diversified technique as well as many other techniques including manipulation under anesthesia. Dr. Bloom has worked with various university programs to improve overall athletic performance.

Bloom Chiropractic provides a program of care designed to improve physical function to assist athletes in achieving their optimal potential. Bloom Chiropractic provides a program of care designed to achieve ion balance within the body. Dr. Bloom is affiliated with multiple drug rehab facilities, helping with the detox process. Detoxification is one of the purposes of chiropractic care, which is done in order to restore or correct the positive and negative ions in the body.

Bloom Chiropractic is affiliated with multiple ambulatory surgical centers and hospitals around the nation, by bringing their expertise of neuromusculoskeletal health conditions. Bloom Chiropractic analyzes the body for vertebral subluxation(s), a severe form of spine and nerve stress, using analysis tools and then corrects or removes any spinal nerve stress using various spinal adjustment techniques.

Conversation with Dr. Bloom

Question: Tell us a little about Bloom Chiropractic & Wellness Center.

Dr. Bloom: We provide high quality, cost-effective health care that delivers the best value to the people we serve in a positive environment of caring and in association with recognized teaching and research.

We see a wide range of patients from newborns to 100 years young. Anybody we feel we can help through the proper diagnostic workup is a candidate. Chiropractic proposes that segmental dysfunction of the spinal column and other articulations can affect nervous system function and the expression of health, which may result in symptoms, infirmity, and disease.

Bloom Chiropractic makes our patient's health our top priority. We are here to assist in optimizing your health's maximum potential.

We look for subluxation(s) as a cause of symptoms and pain. We've been successful in helping patients with multiple symptoms such as: lower back pain, neck pain, and joint pain including: shoulder, elbow, wrist, hand pain, hip, knee, ankle, foot pain, and much more.

Treatments can also help patients find relief from sciatica, whiplash, herniated discs, migraines and headaches, sports injuries, allergies, and asthma as well as many other benefits.

You might be asking yourself, "How can chiropractors help with so many different issues involving the body?" Dr. Bloom's philosophy, as a chiropractic practitioner, is that once we restore the body's biomechanical function, it allows the nervous system to produce the proper neurological impulse to the organs, glands, muscles, skin dermatome or whatever the end that particular nerve supplies.

Question: Can you explain subluxation?

Dr. Bloom: Subluxation is misalignment or restriction between the structures of the spine. If you're looking at the spine straight on, you want it to be relatively straight. If you look at it from the side view, or lateral view, you want those key lordotic and kyphotic curves to be within normal ranges of motion. The term "subluxation" is used by doctors of chiropractic to depict the altered position of the vertebra and subsequent functional loss, which determines the location for the spinal manipulation."Subluxation" has been defined medically as "...a partial abnormal separation of the articular surfaces of a joint."

Chiropractors have expanded the term to include a complex of functions (i.e., the subluxation complex) as "...an alteration of the biomechanical and physiological dynamics of contiguous structures which can cause neural disturbances."

What we are looking for is any misalignment or subluxation that's putting pressure on the nerves. You want a fully functional nervous system.

Question: Can you go deeper into the role chiropractic care plays in the healing process of these issues?

Dr. Bloom: Actually, we don't cure anything as Chiropractors, however what profession really cures anything? What we do is remove pressure off the nerves from the misalignment in the bones of the spine or in the joints and we assist the body in healing itself.

Here's an analogy: if you cut your finger, how would you treat it? You can get a tetanus shot, penicillin shot, apply an antibiotic cream like Neosporin, apply a Band-Aid, and/or any number of things, and yes, your body's going to heal. However, if you cut a piece of steak and apply the same treatment, it's not going to heal because it's not alive due to no electrical impulse from an active nervous system. So that's what I mean when I say we don't cure anything as chiropractors. Your body does the healing. We simply adjust the spine with a goal of restoring the normal biomechanical function of the joint to assist the body in maximal function, to heal itself.

Bloom Chiropractic patients often express how great they feel after an adjustment. We love to hear this; however we want everyone to fully realize the complete process that takes place through each adjustment. Let us demonstrate this for you using the Safety Pin Cycle.

The Safety Pin Cycle shows the flow of mental impulses through the nerve system from the brain to the body using a safety pin. Your brain is in constant communication to your entire body through your nerve system. The relationship of the vertebrae in your spine determines if your safety pin is connected, a closed safety pin, or disconnected, an open safety pin.

When vertebrae of the spine are not in proper relationship, this causes nerve interference, segmental dysfunction, and your safety pin is disconnected. When vertebrae in your spine are in proper relationship, segmental function, then they are able to protect the vital information traveling through the nerve system and your safety pin is connected.

Every chiropractic adjustment you receive restores the proper relationship of vertebrae, removing any interference in the impulses traveling through the nerve system neurologically connecting your brain to your body and allowing your body's innate intelligence to have optimal control for adaptation. A chiropractic adjustment reconnects your safety pin. Understanding the Safety Pin Cycles means you know chiropractic can work for you. Keep your safety pin closed by visiting Bloom Chiropractic or your local chiropractor for regular spinal checks.

Question: Besides physical relief, what kind of impact can this have on a patient's mental wellness?

Dr. Bloom: Of course, increasing flexibility, range of motion, and decreasing pain would make anybody happier, especially if they've been dealing with pain symptoms or discomfort for an extensive amount of time.

Even patients who have minor pain(s), who live with it, and don't realize the irritationit's causing in their life, it's always beneficial to have an increase in flexibility and decrease of pain. For emotional reasons, for work-related stress, and for musculoskeletal complaints.

Most often people associate chiropractic care with lessening the aches and pains of daily life. These may be caused by frequent exercise, sitting at a desk all day, a past car accident or countless other injury-producing events. But what if that main cause of your daily pain isn't physical, but mental? According the Anxiety and Depression Association of America, major depression at any point in time impacts roughly three to five percent of all people and there is about a 17% lifetime risk of a person developing this condition.

Additionally, roughly a half of all those diagnosed with depression also suffer from anxiety.

While medications are most often prescribed for anxiety and depression, many prefer to take the route of holistic healing, including chiropractic care, which can also assist with these symptoms.

How could chiropractic care help emotional healing?

Here are some interesting facts regarding how chiropractic care can help with mental health as well:

Study Results from the Journal of Upper Cervical Chiropractic Research:

A study designed to test the correlation between chiropractic care and its impact on mental health was published in the Journal of Upper Cervical Chiropractic Research on June 20, 2013. This study cited prior research that showed of the 2818 patients undergoing chiropractic care, 76% reported an improvement in their mental/emotional health. Additionally, these 76% also reported positive changes in stress and increased life enjoyment in the months after receiving chiropractic care. Similar findings have also been reported in the American Journal of Psychiatry. So how can having a properly aligned spine impact your mental health?

How Chiropractic Care Improves Mental Health:

One way that chiropractic care can help mental health is by decreasing any physical pain that may be clouding the mind. As anyone with chronic pain can attest to, this discomfort can have a serious impact on mood and mental health. As the spine becomes aligned and pain decreases, anxiety and depression from pain are proven to lessen throughout treatment. This was further illustrated by a study of participants complaining of anxiety or depression who underwent 12 sessions of chiropractic care. As a result, muscle tension decreased and mental clarity increased as well.

Decreases Chronic Pain, a Common Cause of Depression:

When chronic pain is a part of your daily life, not only is it hard to focus, but suddenly you are no longer feeling well enough to be social and take part in activities you once loved. Studies have proven that depression occurs at a rate of three to four times higher in those with chronic pain when compared to their healthier peers. The cycle of chronic pain and depression can continue on and on unless a positive change is made. Regular chiropractic adjustments have proven to decrease pain, depression, and anxiety and allow for a healthier (mentally and physically) existence.

Changes Misalignments Which Impact the Nervous System:

Our moods are regulated by our body's chemistry. This chemistry in your organs as well as your brain is all regulated by the nervous system. Misalignment of the spine (specifically the first, second, or third vertebrae) can cause pressure in the area of the brainstem, which can cause interference neurologically and chemically. Often people turn to medications that are used to alter their brain chemistry, however those looking for a non-medication therapy often find that re-aligning these vertebrae can do wonders for their mental state.

Question: Can you share a story or two about how patients' lives have changed as a result of chiropractic care?

Dr. Bloom: The first one that comes to mind is a gentleman who was 64. He had a boating accident seven years before his first visit, and needed assistance to walk following the accident. He came to my office with a chief complaint of low back pain with a radiculopathy down the leg. He also stated that he experienced dizziness, vertigo, and headaches. After a thorough diagnostic workup, I found a few misalignments that were consistent with the chief complaints and clinical findings. We did see a 2mm herniated disc at segment L4/5 shown on his MRI. After we made sure he was a chiropractic candidate, I adjusted his body, including his upper cervicals (neck). Following the adjustment, he stood up on his own. After further testing, he walked out of the office with no assistance. I think this is pretty significant. His son who helped assist him from for the last seven years was also grateful and intrigued by chiropractic care. It's amazing what your body can accomplish when it is functioning properly.

Another case is a 17-year-old male who visited my office with a chief complaint of pain in his lower neck and upper back. He stated that he had asthma since the age of 10. He was also experiencing severe headaches. After the proper diagnostic workup, and co-managing with his Primary Care Physician "PCP", we adjusted his thoracics and upper cervicals to help ease the headaches, neck, and upper back pain. His pain significantly decreased over a two month duration of treatments, and he stated that he didn't't need to use his inhaler as much as before the chiropractic adjustments. After following up with him one year later, he proudly stated that he was asthma-free. However, we do have to watch for misalignment, just to make sure the symptoms don't return.

Life is an ongoing experience, I recommend getting a "spinal checkup", once a month for segmental dysfunction.

Every form of healing has its time and place. We have a thousand different diagnoses and diseases out there. They are all the result of one thing: stress. If you put enough stress on the chain and on the system, then one of the links won't function properly.

Our philosophy is that the creation of disease is present to give us feedback, or to let us know we have an imbalanced perspective. So the body's signs and symptoms are not something terrible, they are an indicator that we need to address something in our body and/or our lives. We all come with a built in basic program. It's called, self-healing. You get a wound, it regenerates. You get a bacterial infection, the immune system comes and takes care of those bacteria and heals. The immune system is made to heal itself. In fact, parts of the body are literally replaced every day. For example, red blood cells take an estimated time of 120 days to regenerate; the heart and lung tissues take an estimated time of 6 months, and for your entire body, an estimated time of seven years. We need to make sure the nervous system is free of interference or segmental dysfunction to achieve maximal potential for regeneration. Remove physiological stress from the body, and the body does what it is designed to do-it heals itself. I've seen kidneys regenerate. I've seen cancer dissolved. I've seen eyesight improve.

Question: What inspired you to become a chiropractor?

Dr. Bloom: Oh, that's easy. I had neck, back, and right shoulder pain, as well as asthma when I was growing up. I lived with it, with the assistance of inhalers, until my chiropractor adjusted my spine at 15. Following three weeks of chiropractic adjustments, I noticed that I didn't need my inhaler as much. After three months of chiropractic treatments, I asked my Primary Care Physician if I could retest my lungs. He examined me and reviewed my peak flow chart and verified that I only needed an emergency inhaler,

Albuterol. I would go in for checkups every six months until the age of 18, with little to no breathing issues. Without the pain and inhalers, I could pursue my career in volleyball. I played division I at Southern Mississippi, and I don't think I would have been able to do that without chiropractic. After I graduated, I went on to Chiropractic College to pay it forward. I was happy to pay it forward to the 17-year-old young man when I did, as well as other patients.

Question: What would you say to someone who feels medication is the only treatment for issues like asthma?

Dr. Bloom: Well, I think there's a time and a place for everything. I didn't know about chiropractors or if I was a candidate for them at the time. I've had to visit the ER a few times from the age of eight to 15, for severe asthma attacks when the inhalers weren't enough relief. Therefore, I am absolutely thankful for medication and those doctors who helped me during that time. They gave me the proper prescriptions, with a goal breathing more efficiently, and all was well. Later on, I learned about chiropractic, and over time, approximately three months of care, I did not need my inhaler; however I received chiropractic adjustments due to tight muscles and segmental dysfunction.

Question: What are some common fears that might prevent someone from seeking chiropractic care?

Dr. Bloom: "Is it going to hurt?" It's not unusual to get nervous whenever someone touches your neck. Located in your neck is a brain stem spinal cord that is encapsulated by the vertebrae and you having vital nerve flow throughout your spine and body. I recommend that you make sure that whoever is assisting you with your body is trained and credentialed to perform the appropriate protocols needed for your treatment. People get a little nervous due to the audible or noises a chiropractic adjustment can make. It requires good rapport between the doctor and patient. However, that's why there are different techniques. If you don't feel comfortable with one, then another should work for you.

We help them overcome this fear during their exam by asking for two short-term and two long-term goals. One short-term and one long-term goal pertaining to their pain levels, and what they plan to do with their body to achieve their lifestyle goals.

Do what you love. If you don't know what brings you love or joy, ask, "What is my joy? What do I love?" As you commit to what you love or what brings you joy, you will attract an avalanche of joyful things that you love because you are radiating love and joy.

The other goals focus on the activities they'd like to do, so we can address them, and give them some motivation. For example, I had one patient that wanted to be able to throw a baseball around with his grandson, but he was having shoulder issues, and he couldn't't lift his arm past 35 degrees abduction. We achieved his goal of 180 degrees abduction, and he stated that he played baseball, and threw catch with his grandson after 20 visits of chiropractic care. The goals are so that you can live your life the way you want to live it with maximum biomechanical function.

Another case, a 43-year-old male who couldn't extends his neck or look up. He was set at five degrees flexion for what he claimed was 10 years. It took seven weeks of chiropractic care so that he could look up at 45 degrees extension. He started lifting weights because I, as well as the other Primary Care Physician "PCP" approved. Both upper extremities increased in diameter, which is a huge improvement, because due to the diminished impulse prior to his first visit, he was having issues with increasing the right arm muscular strength. He was very satisfied with the results.

We couldn't't continue care due to him moving; however we all were satisfied with the results. I then referred him to a chiropractor in his city to continue his treatment plan.

Question: What lesson did you learn early on that still impacts how you operate Bloom Chiropractic & Wellness Center?

Dr. Bloom: I learned many lessons just by watching and practicing. The treatment plan is time efficient, which helps our patients get back to their life's activities. I do try to motivate them, but not push them too hard, because people are going to do what they feel comfortable or capable of doing. I never want to push anything, and cause a strain or delay in treatment. Our goal to assist them by being positive, and motivational while utilizing an effective treatment plan. I have learned that chiropractic treatments combined with positive motivation, presents the best outcomes in my experience as a practitioner.

Another lesson I've learned is to always do what I think will lead to the best outcome for the patient. Always give them a few different options, and allow them time to research their condition so that they can make their own decisions, and feel confident in their treatment plan.

I learned this by working with hospitals and ambulatory surgical centers, watching how different specialties work, and seeing the outcomes of the patients. Most of their stress is due to a combination of pain, fear, and anxiety. We motivate with a positive attitude and a reputable healthcare team for our patients.

Question: What's the one thing we haven't covered that you want to share with someone who is considering chiropractic?

Dr. Bloom: We stay focused, and disciplined so that we can give our patients 100%. People are happy to get adjusted because they see the progress after the first few visits. People are happy to achieve better results, and see progress. They come back for maintenance about once a month, and get treated on their birthdays, and other holidays. People also fly in to visit Bloom Chiropractic for their chiropractic adjustment, including overseas. Other countries aren't as fortunate as we are to have the healthcare system we offer. Patients see the benefits of chiropractic. Our goal at Bloom Chiropractic is to make sure their day is better after they walk through the doors.

Question: How can someone find out more about Bloom Chiropractic and Wellness Center?

Dr. Bloom: You can find more information about Bloom Chiropractic at www.bloomchirohouston.com, www.bloomchirop.com, Facebook, Twitter, LinkedIn, and YouTube as well as many other avenues. I also perform manipulations under anesthesia in various states. If anyone has questions about the pain they are experiencing or about their general health, they can contact the office at 832.930.2261,or they can email us at info@bloomchirop.com or admin@bloomchirop.com.They can also follow our YouTube videos.I have a "Stretching and Strengthening" series on YouTube where they can work out with me. I break it down for beginners, intermediates, and experts, of all ages. We also have techniques for people who need wheelchair assistance. We see many different conditions from people who need wheelchair assistance tothose who use prosthetics, have spinal fusions, orthotic implants, or patients who have minor aches and pains. Chiropractic can be for everybody!

www.ingramcontent.com/pod-product-compliance
Lightning Source LLC
Chambersburg PA
CBHW070518200326
41519CB00013B/2846